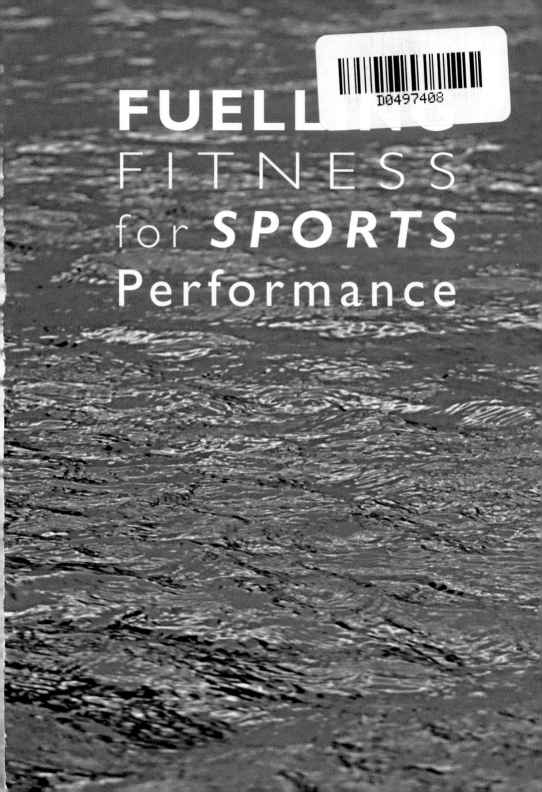

FUELLING
FITNESS
for *SPORTS*
Performance

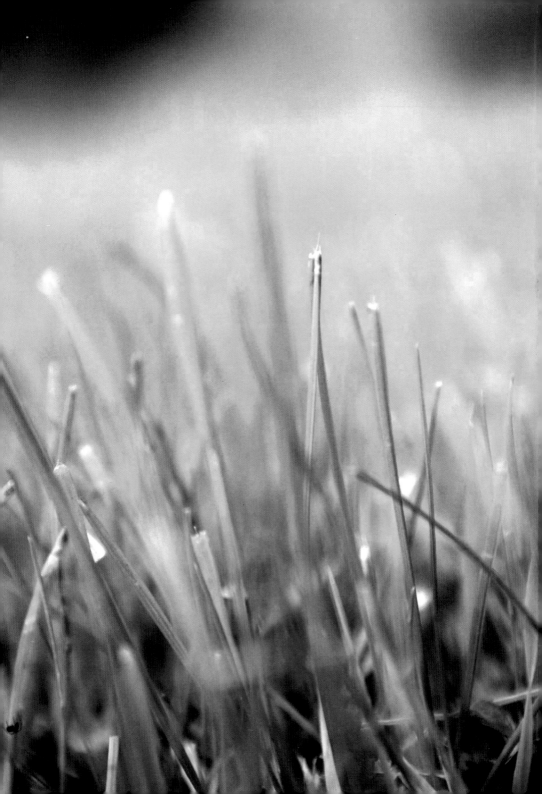

FUELLING
FITNESS
for *SPORTS*
Performance

SPORTS NUTRITION GUIDE

Dr Samantha Stear

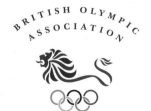

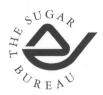

Published by The Sugar Bureau:
The Sugar Bureau, Duncan House, Dolphin Square, London SW1V 3PW, UK

In association with The British Olympic Association:
The British Olympic Association, 1 Wandsworth Plain, London SW18 1ET, UK

British Library Cataloguing in Publication Data.
A catalogue record for this book is available from the British Library.

ISBN 0-9501443-1-2

Note: Whilst every effort has been made to ensure that the content of this book
       is technically accurate and sound, neither the author nor the publishers can accept
       responsibility for any injury or loss sustained as a result of the use of this material.

       None of the athletes/individuals pictured are meant in any way to endorse the foods or
       supplements that are being discussed in the text and are present for illustrative purposes only.

Printed and bound in Great Britain by Fisherprint Ltd, Peterborough, Cambs.

Acknowledgements

Many thanks to such a fantastic and supportive team

Sports Science Consultant	Professor Ronald Maughan
Sports Dietitian Consultants	Jeanette Crosland Penny Hunking
Editorial Team	Dr Richard Cottrell Anna Wheeler Dr Samantha Stear
Designer	Paul Margiotta
Food Photography	Philip Reeson
Sports Photography	Courtesy of Getty Images
with additional contributions from	*Philip Reeson Grant Pritchard Ronald Maughan Craig Nottingham*

Fuelling Fitness for Sports Performance is based on the conclusions of the *International Olympic Committee (IOC) Consensus Conference on Sports Nutrition 2003*. We gratefully acknowledge all the scientific experts who contributed to the conference and the resulting manuscripts.

Sam would also like to thank the team of specialized sports dietitians for all their excellent contributions. In addition, there have been many others who have put a lot of effort and encouragement into producing this book and in particular I would like to thank my husband Craig; Richard Budgett, Nick Fellows and Greg Whyte from the British Olympic Association; Brendan Kemp at Getty Images; and all the crew at the Sugar Bureau - Ali, Anna, Jenny, Jo & Richard.

The production of *Fuelling Fitness for Sports Performance* was supported by an educational grant from The Sugar Bureau.

Contents

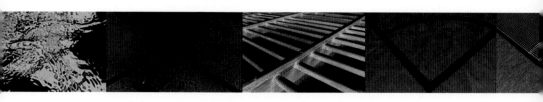

Contributors

Jacqueline Boorman
RD ASD
Accredited Sports Dietitian
www.diet-coaching.com

Jeanette Crosland
MSc RD ASD
Accredited Sports Dietitian
Nutrition Consultant to the
BOA and BPA

Jane Griffin
BSc RD ASD RNutr
Accredited Sports Dietitian
and Nutrition Consultant
www.eatwellperformbetter.co.uk

Marianne Hayward
SRD ASD
Accredited Sports Dietitian
Member of the Scottish Sports
Dietitians Network

Elaine Hibbert-Jones
BSc SRD ASD
Accredited Sports Dietitian
Chief Diabetes Dietitian

Gill Horgan
RD ASD
Accredited Sports Dietitian
and Consultant Nutritionist
gill.horgan@tesco.net

Penny Hunking
RD ASD RPHNutr
Accredited Sports Dietitian
and Nutrition Consultant
www.energise.co.uk

Wendy Martinson
RD ASD
Consultant Dietitian and
Accredited Sports Dietitian
wendy.martinson@lineone.net

Jan Masson
SRD ASD
Accredited Sports Dietitian
Member of the Scottish Sports
Dietitians Network

Gill Regan
MSc SRD ASD
Accredited Sports Dietitian
Chief Paediatric Diabetes Dietitian

Karen Reid
BSc RD ASD
Accredited Sports Dietitian
Works with English Institute
of Sport & UK Athletics
www.performancefood.co.uk

Samantha Stear
PhD MSc BSc RPHNutr
Registered Sport
and Exercise Nutritionist
Science Director,
The Sugar Bureau, UK
www.sugar-bureau.co.uk

Foreword

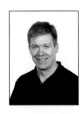

Dr Richard Budgett OBE
Director of Medical Services, British Olympic Association.

This book covers all the important aspects of diet for any individuals who are exercising on a regular basis. Everyone from the recreational athlete to the Olympic champion will find this authoritative book interesting and useful. The chapters cover basic nutrition and then go into detail on controversial topics such as supplements and the proportion of the main constituents of the diet.

Different sports have different requirements and these are covered by experts from appropriate sports. The differing requirements of disabled, diabetic or female athletes are also revealed.

Practical strategies on meal ideas, kit bag snacks and how to record your own food and drink to work out how much carbohydrate, protein and fat your diet provides, helps turn the theory into practice. Plus, any individual who reads and uses this book can be confident that their diet and nutrition is optimum for both their health and performance.

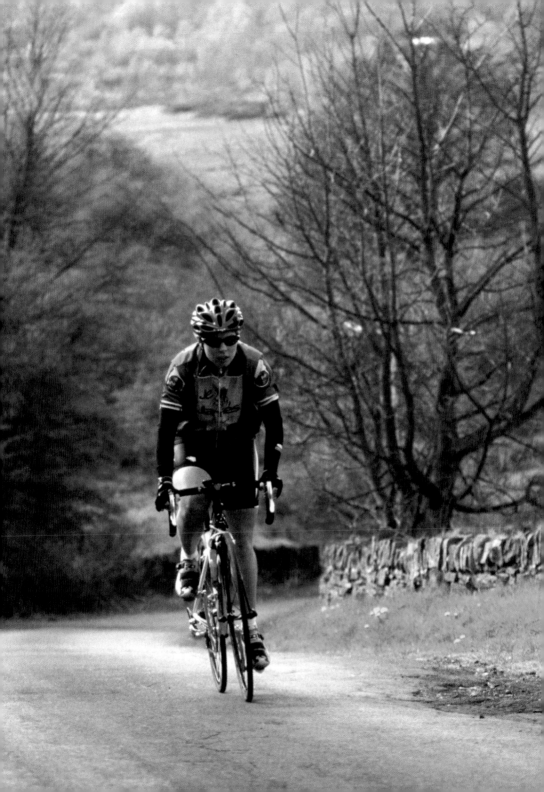

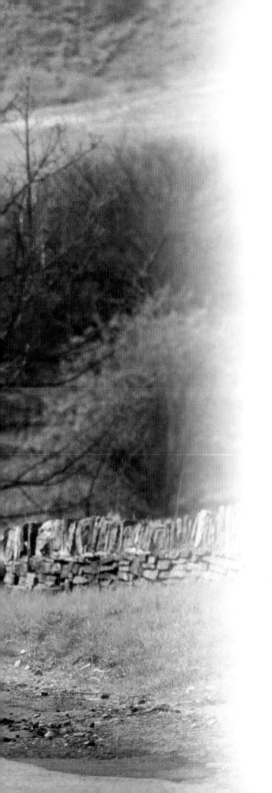

Introduction

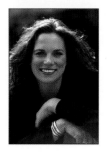

Dr Samantha Stear PhD MSc BSc RPHNutr
is a Registered Sport and Exercise Nutritionist and fully qualified fitness consultant and trainer. Sam has a biomedical science degree from University College London, a masters degree in nutrition from King's College London, and a PhD from Cambridge University. Sam has competed in various sports at both national and international levels, and maintains a keen interest in sports performance and the well-being of athletes. She is a regular contributor to the consumer and professional media on topics concerning health, nutrition and exercise.

Fuelling Fitness for Sports Performance has been written to bring you the latest that the science of sports nutrition has to offer. In essence it's for anyone who is serious about their training – whether an elite athlete, an active competitor, or someone who simply enjoys getting a buzz from pushing themselves physically. If you want to perform to the best of your ability then you need the best advice.

In June 2003, the top sports nutrition scientists from across the world met to produce a new International Olympic Committee (IOC) Consensus Statement on Sports Nutrition. Thanks to all the contributors involved in the IOC Consensus Meeting, we have been able to bring you this book. We have tried to digest the huge amount of technical information from the IOC manuscripts and present them in a manner that will meet the needs of a wide range of sports and exercise enthusiasts, along with allied professionals such as nutritionists, coaches, physiotherapists and doctors.

I make no excuse if the overall style of the book appears to have a hard edge – it wasn't meant to be 'fluffy'! After all, training is hard – even on those light days when it's 'just another one in the bag'. Anyone who says training isn't hard either isn't training seriously or is lying!

Life in the world of sport revolves around training and competition. To strive for performance improvements – be it skill, power, strength, speed or endurance – you need to put the training in! Food isn't a magic bullet – it can't make you throw the javelin another metre, serve more aces, or knock seconds off your personal best! But, your diet is absolutely central in supporting your training to make it possible.

Competing is a bit like any other exam or test – what you don't know or haven't practiced by the time it gets to the competition is more or less too late! So you need to get your preparation right – both mentally and physically. Something that I learnt from a coach and its stuck with me ever since is the '6 Ps':

Prior **P**reparation and **P**lanning **P**revents a **P**oor **P**erformance

There are a multitude of factors involved in preparation that are all intrinsically linked - some you can change, some you can't! For instance, 'Does the person choose the sport or does the sport choose the person?' Maybe this question will never be answered, but without a doubt, genetics – or natural talent - has a huge role to play. In sport size does matter – rowers benefit from long levers and jockeys from a small, light frame. But simply being born isn't going to make you into an Olympic Champion. There's a lot more hard work, and not forgetting motivation, to get you there.

So although you need all the pieces of the jigsaw to complete the picture, nutrition has an essential role to play. Get your diet right and it'll fuel your training to help you reach your goals. In *Fuelling Fitness for Sports Performance,* we delve into all the key dietary issues to help you fuel your training and recover ready for the next work-out. But, it's not about rules and we won't tell you exactly what to do! What we hope it does is give you the science to empower you to make better decisions.

It's important to remember that any competitive edge, be it from nutrition, training tactics, equipment or some other variable, even if it only produces the tiniest of additional advantages, is highly beneficial! After all, it could help you achieve a personal best or perhaps make the difference between winning an Olympic Gold and not qualifying!

Fuelling Training, Fuelling Fitness, Fuelling Sport.....
Whatever your goal - fuel-up and go!

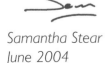

Samantha Stear
June 2004

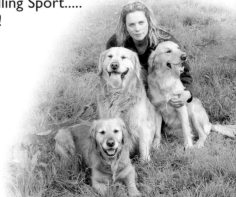

Key Messages

- Life in the world of sport revolves around training and competition. To be able to sustain training, as well as strive for performance improvements – be it skill, power, strength, speed or endurance – you need to be able to recover between one training session and the next.

- A healthy balanced diet is essential for long-term good health. Whatever your sport or fitness programme, you can optimize your training to reach your goals by making informed dietary choices. Good food choices help ensure fuel needs are met to promote adaptations to training, to help you recover quickly to continue and intensify training, and to ensure good health to prevent illness and injury.

- A varied, well-balanced diet, that meets the energy demands of training, should provide adequate amounts of all the essential nutrients. It is vital to get your energy intake right – too much or too little and health and performance are at risk. The right diet will help you achieve the optimal body size and build for your sport, and the optimal mix of fuel stores, to enhance exercise performance.

- Carbohydrate is the key nutrient for energy supply. Make carbohydrate-rich foods the focus of your diet. The more intense your training programme, the more carbohydrates you need to eat. The body's carbohydrate stores are relatively small so need to be topped-up regularly to supply and restock fuel for training. Nutrient-rich carbohydrate snacks and meals provide a good source of protein and other nutrients.

- ¤ Protein plays an important role in building and repairing muscle. Providing energy needs are met, a varied diet is likely to supply more than enough protein. Well chosen vegetarian and vegan diets can also meet protein needs.

- ¤ Maintaining adequate hydration is important for exercise performance. How much fluid you need depends on how hard you work, how long you exercise and the environmental conditions. Try to drink fluid at a rate that limits fluid losses – don't lose more than 1-2% of body weight and don't drink so much that you gain weight during exercise. To effectively restore hydration levels after exercise you'll need to replace both water and salts in excess of the fluid losses.

- ¤ Indiscriminate use of supplements is unwise due to potential health, contamination, and doping risks.

- ¤ Effective recovery requires rest, restocking carbohydrate stores and replacing fluid and salt losses.

- ¤ Plan and practise fuelling, hydrating and recovery strategies during training – don't try anything new during important competitions! When training or competing away from home, be prepared by taking a range of high carbohydrate meals and snacks with you.

- ¤ This book brings you the latest scientific information on sports nutrition, but it is no substitute for advice from a qualified professional. Athletes will benefit from the guidance of a qualified sports nutrition expert, to help develop personalized dietary plans that are sport and environment specific, and tailored to meet their individual needs and preferences.

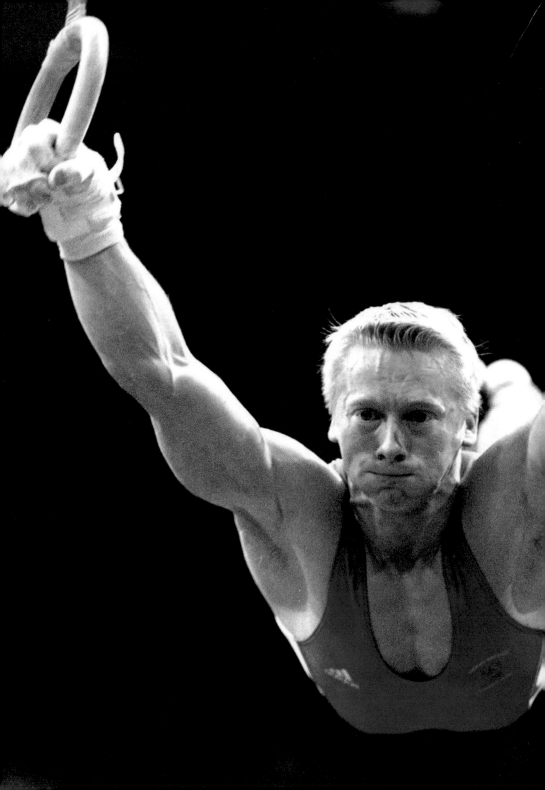

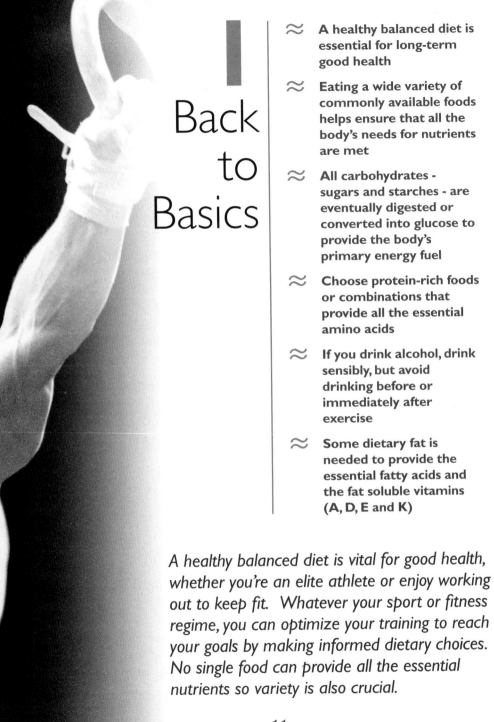

Back to Basics

≈ **A healthy balanced diet is essential for long-term good health**

≈ **Eating a wide variety of commonly available foods helps ensure that all the body's needs for nutrients are met**

≈ **All carbohydrates - sugars and starches - are eventually digested or converted into glucose to provide the body's primary energy fuel**

≈ **Choose protein-rich foods or combinations that provide all the essential amino acids**

≈ **If you drink alcohol, drink sensibly, but avoid drinking before or immediately after exercise**

≈ **Some dietary fat is needed to provide the essential fatty acids and the fat soluble vitamins (A, D, E and K)**

A healthy balanced diet is vital for good health, whether you're an elite athlete or enjoy working out to keep fit. Whatever your sport or fitness regime, you can optimize your training to reach your goals by making informed dietary choices. No single food can provide all the essential nutrients so variety is also crucial.

11

The key to making our diet healthy and balanced is to ensure it provides adequate energy from the consumption of a wide variety of commonly available foods, so that we can meet our carbohydrate, protein and fat needs for both health and exercise. The food we eat provides the nutrients required by the body. However, no one food or food group can provide all the essential nutrients the body needs for good health, so eating a wide variety including plenty of fruit and vegetables is also key to ensuring an adequate supply of vitamins, minerals and dietary fibre. (Vitamins and minerals are covered separately in chapter 6)

The body's energy supply is derived from the nutrients in our diet. Nutrients are found in differing amounts in foods and are broken down in the body to provide a certain quantity of energy, which is commonly expressed as kilocalories (kcal) per gram (g). The main energy-yielding nutrients in our diet are:

- Carbohydrate 3.75 kcal/g
- Protein 4 kcal/g
- Alcohol 7 kcal/g
- Fat 9 kcal/g

Carbohydrates

Dietary carbohydrate is provided by a wide variety of carbohydrate-rich food and drinks. However, all carbohydrates - both sugars and starches - are ultimately converted to and absorbed into the blood in the form of glucose, to provide the primary energy fuel. There is no universal system that can adequately describe the diverse metabolic, functional and nutritional features of the various carbohydrate foods. One of the simplest ways of classifying carbohydrates is by their structure. Basically, they can be divided into three main groups:

1. Monosaccharides

These are single molecules of sugar. The monosaccharides are:

- Glucose
- Fructose
- Galactose

Glucose is found in most carbohydrate foods including sugars and starches. All carbohydrates are eventually digested or converted into glucose. Fructose is also known as fruit sugar and is found in fruits, vegetables and honey.

It is converted into glucose by the liver. Galactose is part of lactose, the sugar found in milk.

2. Disaccharides

These are two linked sugar molecules which are broken down into the monosaccharides by digestion. The disaccharides are:

- Sucrose = glucose + fructose

- Lactose = glucose + galactose

- Maltose = glucose + glucose

Sucrose (table sugar) normally comes from sugar beet and cane, but is also found naturally in all fruits and vegetables, and even most herbs and spices. Lactose is found in milk and milk products. Maltose is formed when starch is broken down.

3. Starches

Starch (polysaccharide) is simply hundreds of molecules of glucose sugar joined together. When starch is digested, it is first broken down into maltose and then into glucose.

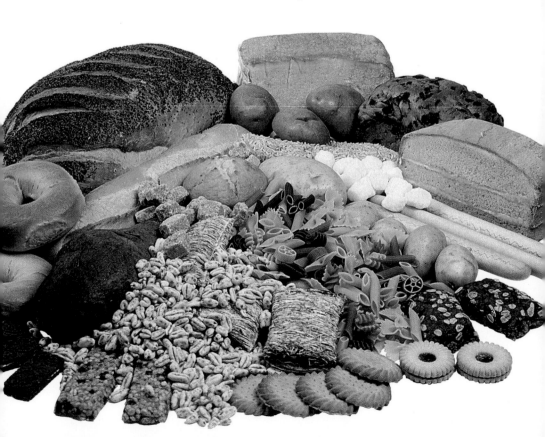

So, as you can see, the major difference between sugars and starches is the size of the molecule. Nonetheless, foods containing significant amounts of carbohydrates have been classed according to the major type of carbohydrate they contain. This has led to the simplistic division of carbohydrate-containing foods into 'simple' (mainly consisting of sugars) and 'complex' (mainly consisting of starches). This over-simplification is confusing as the majority of naturally occurring foods contain a mixture of sugars and starches, as well as other nutrients.

Furthermore, as most carbohydrates will ultimately end-up as glucose to provide that vital energy fuel, one type is not necessarily better than the other. Consequently, several other factors may be more important to athletes, including how rapidly the carbohydrate is converted to glucose, alongside issues such as appeal and practicality, which may often be specific to the individual and the exercise situation. Further information about the carbohydrate content of foods, and the amount - and in some situations the type - of carbohydrate your training programme needs can be found in the section on fuelling training and recovery.

Protein

Protein is essential for life and is a major part of the body. Throughout the day there is a continual process of protein turnover, with proteins being broken down and formed at the same time. The largest reservoir of protein is found in the muscles, but there is a limited capacity to store new proteins. Therefore, protein intake in excess of requirements is either broken down to provide energy or stored as fat or carbohydrate.

Protein is needed for the growth and repair of tissues. During digestion, proteins are broken down into smaller units called amino acids. There are about 20 different naturally occurring amino acids, which can be combined to make a vast array of different proteins. Our bodies can make proteins from amino acids, but we are unable to produce nine of the amino acids - the essential amino acids - so these must be supplied in adequate amounts by the diet. The semi-essential amino acids can be made in the body, providing certain essential amino acids are present in the diet in sufficient amounts e.g. cysteine needs methionine and tyrosine needs phenylalanine. (See Table 1)

Table 1. Amino acids

Essential
Histidine
Isoleucine
Leucine
Lysine
Methionine
Phenylalanine
Threonine
Tryptophan
Valine
Semi-essential
Cysteine
Tyrosine
Non-essential
Alanine
Arginine (essential in infants)
Aspartic acid (also as asparagine)
Glutamic acid (also as glutamine)
Glycine
Proline
Serine

Only some foods - the complete protein foods - contain all the essential amino acids. In general, foods from animal sources contain substantial amounts of all the essential amino acids, but foods from other sources can be combined with each other to make complete protein foods. For example, the protein quality of plant products is improved when dairy products are added to a plant food and when plant-based foods, such as wheat and beans, are mixed together. Table 2 gives some examples of protein-rich foods or combinations that provide all the essential amino acids in sufficient amounts.

Protein combining is not necessary in a vegetarian diet where milk, cheese and eggs are eaten, because these foods provide adequate amounts of all the essential amino acids. Strict vegetarians, and in particular vegans who eat no dairy products or eggs, need to plan their diet carefully to ensure that their combination of plant foods provides them with all the essential amino acids. However, this mixing and matching of plant foods to provide all the essential amino acids, does not need to occur at the same meal but can take place over the course of the day.

Table 2. Complete protein foods

Type	Examples
Dairy products	Milk, yoghurt
Eggs	Boiled, scrambled, omelette
Fish	Fresh or tinned e.g. salmon, tuna
Meat and meat products	Beef, lamb, ham, sausages
Poultry	Chicken, turkey
Grains plus legumes	Bean curry or lentils with rice, peanut butter sandwich, bread with hummous, baked beans on toast
Grains plus nuts or seeds	Muesli mix with oats and nuts or seeds e.g. hazelnuts or sunflower seeds, rice salad with nuts e.g. walnuts, sesame seed spread (tahini) on bread
Legumes plus nuts or seeds	Mix of peanuts and nuts e.g. cashews
Grains plus dairy products	Breakfast cereal and milk, rice pudding, pizza or pasta with cheese, cheese sandwich
Legumes plus dairy products	Bean curry in a yoghurt based sauce, bean chilli with cheese

Note: legumes include pulses (e.g. peas and beans) and peanuts

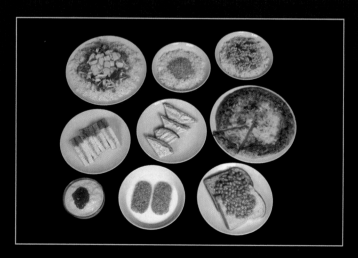

Complete protein food combinations

The protein content of foods and protein needs for training are covered specifically in the section on protein. Special considerations regarding vegetarian athletes are also discussed in chapter 9.

Alcohol

The advice on sensible drinking exists to limit the health risks associated with excessive intakes of alcohol. In the long-term, continued heavy drinking causes liver damage and other health problems. In the short-term, excessive amounts of alcohol can be toxic to the individual as well as potentially dangerous to others, due to the resulting loss of co-ordination or self-control and behavioural changes. It's also important to rehydrate properly after exercise before drinking alcohol as it can cause dehydration and slow down the recovery process. (See section on fuelling training and recovery)

Furthermore, many sports are associated with muscle damage and soft tissue injuries, either directly due to the exercise or from the tackling and collisions involved in contact sports. Although the evidence is limited, it would be advisable for athletes who suffer considerable muscle damage and soft tissue injuries to avoid alcohol in the immediate recovery phase - probably best avoided for 24 hours following the event.

Alcohol is generally no longer a banned substance in sport. However, it is still considered banned in some sports such as fencing and shooting. It is likely that its consumption will interfere with skilled performance in sport, and, in particular may increase the risk of injury. Likewise, it is illegal to drive following the consumption of moderate to large amounts of alcohol due to the interference with the judgement and skill required to drive safely.

Therefore guidelines for sensible drinking should be followed at all times and especially in the period after training or competition. In the UK 1 unit is defined as 8g of alcohol and is roughly equivalent to the alcohol content of:

- a single 25ml measure of spirits e.g. gin, vodka, whisky, brandy

- a 50ml measure of sherry or fortified wine such as port

- a small (100ml) glass of wine

- half a pint of standard strength (3.5% alcohol) beer, lager or cider

Based on the evidence of associated health risks the recommended maximum levels of alcohol consumption were originally set at no more than 21 units per week for men and 14 units per week for women. However, following the growing evidence of the detrimental effects on health of heavy or 'binge' drinking, the sensible drinking guidelines were switched to daily maximum intakes. These guidelines state that maximum daily intakes should not exceed 3-4 units for men and 2-3 units for women. In addition, alcohol intake during pregnancy should not exceed 1 unit per day.

It's also important to remember that alcohol is a high-energy (provides 7 kcal per gram) and nutrient-poor food, and consequently its intake should be limited so that it neither displaces other nutrients nor results in unnecessary increases in body fat.

Fat

Although the excessive consumption of dietary fat is discouraged this doesn't mean that we need to become fat phobic. It's necessary that we include some fat in our diet to provide us with both the essential fatty acids and the fat soluble vitamins - A, D, E and K.

Table 3. Good sources of essential fatty acids

Omega-3
Oily fish e.g. salmon, mackerel, sardines, herring, pilchards, and tuna in oil
Linseeds and pumpkin seeds
Oils e.g. soyabean and rapeseed
Walnuts
Sweet potato
Omega-6
Seeds e.g. sunflower and sesame
Nuts
Oils e.g. sunflower, safflower, corn, groundnut, sesame, rapeseed and soya oils
Polyunsaturated margarine

Additionally, some fat is stored within the muscles and can be used as an energy source - see the sections on fuelling training and recovery and optimizing competition performance.

Furthermore, avoiding all foods that contain more than a trace of fat reduces the variety of foods in the diet, and, in extreme cases, could lead to nutrient deficiencies. For example, dairy products are often avoided due to being 'too high in fat', but they are a valuable source of protein, calcium and many other vitamins and minerals. Besides, if fat intake needs to be restricted there are plenty of low-fat options.

Dietary fat is composed of three kinds of fatty acids:

- Saturated fatty acids (SFA)
- Monounsaturated fatty acids (MUFA)
- Polyunsaturated fatty acids (PUFA)

A typical dietary fat contains a mixture of both saturated and unsaturated (MUFA and PUFA) fatty acids. Different foods have varying proportions of fatty acids such that the fat in meat, dairy products and coconuts is predominantly SFA; olive and rapeseed oils have a high proportion of MUFA; and sunflower and soya oils are mostly PUFA. Essential fatty acids (EFA) are a sub group of PUFA that our bodies cannot make and therefore they need to be supplied in adequate amounts by the diet. EFA can be divided into 2 classes - the omega-3 (η-3) and omega-6 (η-6) fatty acids. Table 3 gives examples of foods that are good sources of the essential fatty acids.

Dietary intake of omega-6 PUFA needs to be adequate but not excessive, as they potentially lower 'protective' HDL cholesterol levels. Therefore the dietary focus should be on sources rich in omega-3 PUFA. For health, it is recommended that we aim to consume two portions of fish per week, with preferably one of these being oily fish to ensure an adequate supply of omega-3 EFA.

The type of fat that dominates the diet depends on the proportion of different fatty acids present in the choice of foods consumed. Moderate fat diets, where the fat is predominantly supplied by MUFA and PUFA, and SFA are kept low, have been shown to reduce total cholesterol levels, and in particular reduce the levels of the 'harmful' LDL cholesterol. Although, very low fat diets will also achieve this result, the downside is that they also tend to reduce the levels of the 'protective' HDL cholesterol. Foods that are rich in the unsaturated fatty acids include: olive and rapeseed oils; avocados; nuts; sunflower, sesame and pumpkin seeds; and oily fish.

The amount of dietary fat needed depends on several factors including age, body size and training levels. If you need to reduce your fat intake then there are several simple adjustments you can make - opt for lower-fat versions such as semi-skimmed milk; cook by grilling instead of frying; select leaner cuts of meat and trim-off any visible fats.

Increasing your intake of carbohydrate foods - both starches and sugars - has also been shown to help lower dietary fat intake - and of course reduces calorie intake too. However, be careful not to overload your bread, potatoes and pasta with lots of butter, cheese or cream as that would make it high-fat again!

Food labelling on pre-packaged foods will also help if you need to choose 'low' or 'reduced' fat options. All such choices are likely to be better than the full-fat version, but it's important to understand what the terminology means:

- Reduced fat - contains at least 25% less than the standard product

- Low fat - contains less than 3g fat per 100g or 100ml (less than 3%)

- Fat free - contains less than 0.15g fat per 100g or 100ml (less than 0.15%)

However care is still needed as calories still count. Some reduced fat foods such as sausages still contain a considerable amount of fat and calories. Plus it doesn't mean you can forget about portion sizes altogether - just because it's lower in fat doesn't mean you can eat as much as you like!

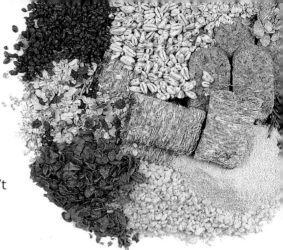

	TEN TOP TIPS TO EAT HEALTHILY
1.	Enjoy your food - healthy eating is not about good or bad foods
2.	Eat a wide variety of different foods
3.	Eat the right amount of energy for your individual needs
4.	Eat more carbohydrates - especially the cereal and starchy sources
5.	Eat at least five portions of fruit and vegetables a day
6.	Eat less fat and replace saturated with unsaturated fats
7.	Avoid adding extra fat and oils to food
8.	Eat moderate amounts of protein
9.	Eat two portions of fish a week - one portion should be oily fish
10.	If you drink alcohol, drink sensibly

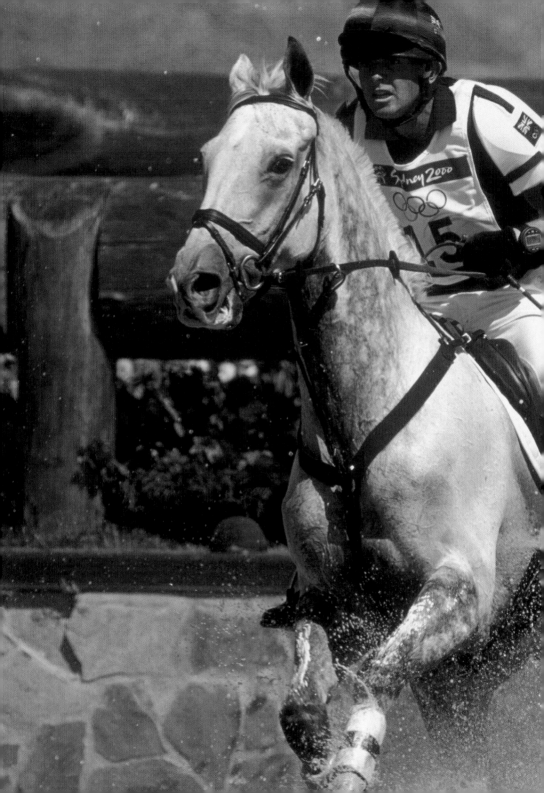

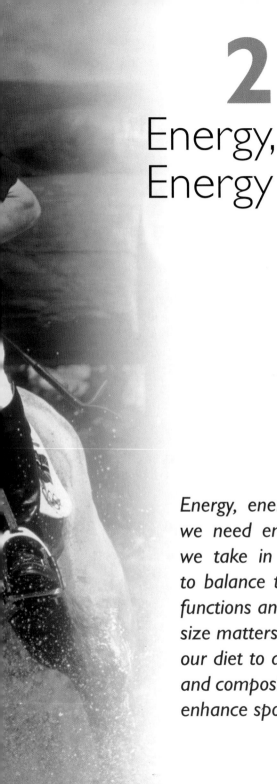

2
Energy, Energy

≈ **You need the correct amount of energy - too much or too little and health and performance are at risk**

≈ **Body weight is not a reliable indicator of either energy balance or macronutrient (carbohydrate, protein and fat) balance**

≈ **Achieving a sport-specific optimal body size, body composition and mix of fuel stores will maximize exercise performance**

≈ **Reproductive disorders in athletes may be caused by low energy availability and not by the stress of exercise**

Energy, energy - whatever we're doing we need energy. But does the energy we take in from food and drink need to balance the energy we use for bodily functions and exercise? After all, in sport, size matters! So how can we manipulate our diet to achieve the optimal body size and composition, and mix of fuel stores, to enhance sport performance?

Whatever we're doing, our bodies require energy. But when we exercise, we need to be able to draw on more of it - faster. As a result, total dietary energy intake needs to be increased to compensate for the energy used up during training. However, many athletes, particularly females and individuals who compete in endurance and aesthetic sports, and sports with weight categories, do not adequately compensate for the energy they use and so end-up constantly energy deficient. In sports where a low body weight is advantageous, many athletes practice extreme weight loss techniques, which in-turn place reproductive and skeletal health, as well as performance, at risk. Consequently, in these sports, there seems to be a great risk of low energy availability. Therefore, it's vital that we get our energy intake right. Too much and body fat increases. But too little and our health and performance are at risk. So where does energy come from?

All the energy needed for exercise comes ultimately from the food and drinks we take in. Part of this energy is used straight away but most is stored for later use. Fat is stored as fat, protein as protein, but carbohydrate is converted to glucose and then stored as glycogen.

Energy Systems

The body uses different energy systems for different types of activity. When we need energy our body breaks up a substance called ATP (adenosine triphosphate) - a high energy molecule consisting of three phosphates attached by energy bonds to adenosine. Energy is released by breaking off a phosphate from ATP to form ADP (adenosine diphosphate). This is a continual cycle - with ADP being converted back into ATP. Three systems in the body create ATP energy. These systems work simultaneously but the contribution from each depends on the type of exercise - its intensity and duration.

1. ATP-CP
The sprint system - provides enough energy for a 5-6 second sprint - and doesn't require oxygen (anaerobic). CP (creatine phosphate) is another high energy molecule where the phosphate can be broken off very quickly - releasing energy - and used to convert ADP back to ATP. The muscles don't have a large store of CP so it's used

up fast. Consequently, creatine supplements have become popular in the hope that their use will maximize the body's creatine muscle stores. (See section on supplements)

2. Anaerobic

The high power system - provides energy for a 90 second power burst. This system is the fast anaerobic (without oxygen) breakdown of glucose for energy but only provides two molecules of ATP along with a waste product called lactic acid - too much of this causes muscle fatigue.

3. Aerobic

The endurance system - how long you can keep going depends on how fit you are! This system is the slow aerobic (with oxygen) breakdown of glucose for energy and provides a massive 38 molecules of ATP - that's nearly 20 times more than the anaerobic system! The aerobic system can also use fat to produce ATP energy. Indeed, one of the consequences of endurance training is that it causes the muscles to

use fat more effectively, and thereby help conserve the limited glycogen (carbohydrate) stores.

Energy Fuel

Carbohydrate, fat and protein are the three main energy fuels for exercise. Each of these nutrients are found in differing amounts in foods and are broken down in the body to provide a certain quantity of energy - measured as kilocalories (kcal) per gram (g):

- ◻ Carbohydrate 3.75 kcal/g
- ◻ Protein 4 kcal/g
- ◻ Fat 9 kcal/g

Hence 1g of fat releases more than twice as much energy as 1g of carbohydrate or protein - but this doesn't mean it's the best energy fuel for exercise!

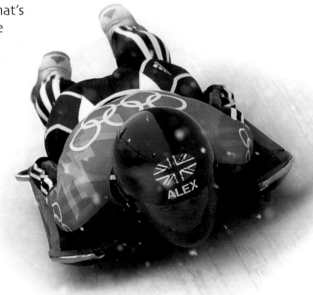

The amount of each fuel - carbohydrate, fat and protein - you use during exercise depends on various factors. The main ones are:

- Type of exercise
- Training intensity
- Duration of work-out
- Frequency of training sessions
- Fitness level
- Dietary intake

Anaerobic activities only use carbohydrate, whereas aerobic activities use all three fuels - although protein is used to a lesser extent than carbohydrate and fat.

During low-intensity exercise, which uses less than 300 kcal each hour, the body uses a greater proportion of fat, a smaller proportion of glucose and fewer calories. As exercise intensity increases, the body gradually uses more glucose and more energy (calories). Therefore, most of the fuel during moderate and high intensity exercise (using more than 500 kcal each hour) will come from glucose.

If you continue to exercise aerobically for a longer period, your body will gradually use more fat and less carbohydrate in an attempt to conserve the limited carbohydrate stores. The fitter you are, the more efficiently your muscles use fat and the longer you can work out.

Consequently, the preferred energy fuel for the muscles is carbohydrate, because it's the only fuel that can power intense exercise for prolonged periods. All carbohydrates - the sugars and starches in the diet - are converted to glucose and stored as glycogen in the muscles and liver. However the body can only store a limited amount. A person weighing 70kg will store around 450g or 1700 kcal of glycogen - at marathon running speed this would keep you going for a couple of hours. So if you want to keep training efficiently you need to keep your glycogen stores topped up. See the section on fuelling training and recovery to discover how much carbohydrate your training programme requires.

Energy Balance

So we need energy to fuel our training programme, but do we always need to be in energy balance? Our daily energy intake from food and drink provides our immediate energy needs - bodily functions, activity and growth - as well as influencing our body's energy stores. The energy stores are also related to exercise performance - they affect our size and physique (body fat and muscle mass), our function, and provide our fuel for exercise.

In sport - size matters! Size is both sport-specific, and in the case of team sports is also often position-specific. For example, sprinters have no use for fat stores (in competition), whereas endurance athletes need them for fuel, swimmers need them for buoyancy and cold-water swimmers need them for insulation! Consequently, many athletes try to manipulate their body size, body composition and fuel stores in an attempt to achieve the characteristics that they believe offer an advantage in their sport. For many, the goal is to reduce body fat while increasing muscle mass and glycogen stores.

In athletes, body weight is not a reliable indicator of either energy or macronutrient (carbohydrate, protein and fat) balance, because it is not able to distinguish between changes in body fat or muscle mass, or to see whether total energy intake provides for optimal fuel stores. Energy balance, in itself, also provides little information about current status or indeed progress towards optimizing body size, body composition and the mix of fuel stores.

Macronutrient Balance

Macronutrients - carbohydrate, protein and fat - are metabolized differently and stored separately. Therefore, carbohydrate, protein and fat intakes and expenditures should also be managed separately to achieve sport-specific body size, composition and energy store objectives. These issues are covered in more detail later on in the book.

In general, excess fats are stored, excess carbohydrate and protein is mostly used up, and alcohol is entirely used up. As discussed above, skeletal muscle fuel selection varies under different exercise conditions, with carbohydrate being preferentially used during short, high-intensity exercise, and fats being preferentially used during prolonged, low-intensity exercise.

So, to lose body fat, you need a negative energy balance and a negative fat balance. This can be created by reducing the intake of fats and increasing the oxidation (burning-up) of fats by exercising. Since lean muscle mass may be increasing as body fat is declining, this may not necessarily involve a reduction in energy intake, energy balance or body weight. Alternatively to increase lean muscle mass, a positive protein balance needs to be created by consuming adequate amounts of complete protein, together with sufficient carbohydrate, as well as undertaking specific muscle-building exercises.

Managing Energy

The energy stores of carbohydrate, protein and fat need to be managed individually. It's important to plan eating strategies according to specific body size and training goals rather than relying on appetite to guide energy and nutritional intake. Individuals should seek advice from a sports nutrition expert such as a sports dietitian or registered sport and exercise nutritionist, to help develop an individual plan, particularly in terms of weight and fat loss strategies.

Athletes should utilize a number of separate biomarkers to monitor their progress towards achieving each of their related goals.

- Body weight (although it is not a reliable or accurate marker of either energy or macronutrient balance and its monitoring can be stressful)

- Skinfold thickness is useful for monitoring changes in body fat stores

- Measurements of changes in muscle strength and endurance are probably the most useful measure of muscle development

- A simple dipstick test for urinary ketones (available from chemists) can provide a marker of inadequate carbohydrate intake

Energy Availability Concerns

Although many athletes reduce their energy intake to assist with body weight and fat loss, it's important that any weight loss takes place sensibly and gradually. Severe restrictions in energy intake are dangerous and can disrupt healthy bodily function.

Some athletes, but particularly females, and those who compete in endurance and aesthetic sports, and sports with weight classes, are constantly energy restricted. For example, surveys show that female endurance athletes - with the exception of cross country skiers - consume about 30% less energy and carbohydrate than male endurance athletes even when body size is accounted for.

This energy restriction impairs performance, growth and health. Metabolic and reproductive disorders in athletes, particularly females, are caused by low energy availability - especially by low carbohydrate availability - and not by the stress of exercise. Energy availability is defined as:

Energy availability
=
total dietary energy intake - energy used in daily activity/exercise

However, neither an eating disorder nor restricted eating is necessary to create reproductive disorders in athletes. Simply expending large amounts of energy in training and failing to compensate this with increased energy intake will disrupt metabolic and reproductive function. It is important to note that less severe reproductive disorders may have no symptoms, for example menstrual regularity may appear to be 'normal' in some females.

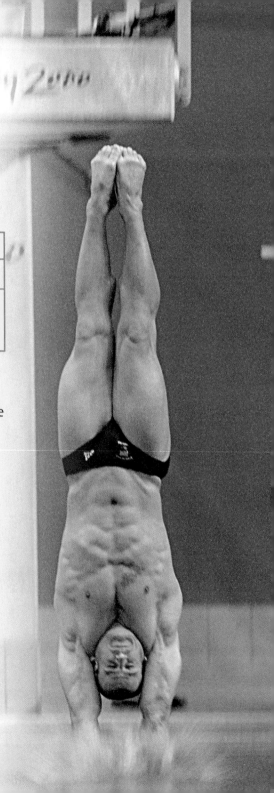

Similar metabolic and reproductive disruptions occur in men, especially those who participate in endurance sports and sports with weight classes. For example, as in energy-deficient female athletes, the reproductive systems in under-nourished male athletes are also suppressed leading to a decline in the level of testosterone. However, without biochemical measurements, problems in male athletes will also often go undetected.

Low energy availability, not the stress of exercise - and neither dietary energy intake nor exercise energy expenditure alone - is what disrupts the metabolic and reproductive systems in men and women.

Athletes can prevent this and restore their reproductive function through dietary change to compensate for exercise energy expenditure without any modification to the training regime - or other stresses. So as long as they are willing to eat they can do all the exercise they like!

There is strong evidence, that in order to protect reproductive and skeletal health, weight loss programmes should avoid energy availability (EA) that falls below 30kcal per kg fat-free mass (FFM) per day. Table 1 shows some examples of low energy availability that fall below the 30kcal per kg of FFM per day.

Table 1. Examples of low energy availability (EA) that fall below the 30kcal per kg of FFM per day:

Athlete description	Dietary energy intake (a)	Energy used in exercise (b)	EA (a-b)	EA/ FFM
Female, 60kg with 20% body fat FFM = 48kg (60 x 0.80) Trains 1.5 hours per day	2100 kcal	800 kcal	1300 kcal	27
Male, 75 kg with 12% body fat FFM = 66kg (75 x 0.88) Trains 2.25 hours per day	3800 kcal	1950 kcal	1850 kcal	28

Female Athlete Triad

Female athletes who suffer disturbances to regular menstrual function are also often found to have sub-optimal bone density. Furthermore, not only is there a higher incidence of stress fractures found in athletes with menstrual dysfunction, but all too often the bone loss in affected individuals is irreversible. Any amenorrhoea (absence of periods) that persists for longer than 6 months without being treated will result in irreversible bone loss.

We lay down bone mineral while we're young until we reach what is known as peak bone mass – the lifetime maximum amount of mineral in our bones – at around 30 years old. In addition, many young athletes are losing bone mineral at a time when they should be accumulating it, and with only a limited time left (until their 30's), peak bone mass is likely to be less than ideal. Losing bone mineral during this 'window of opportunity' can have serious long-term consequences and compromises bone health for life. This can lead to some young athletes having the bone density of a 60 year old. Osteoporosis in a 20 year old athlete is a disaster.

The term 'female athlete triad' has been coined to refer to the three interrelated conditions: disordered eating, amenorrhoea and osteoporosis. Every element of the triad increases the chance of morbidity and mortality, but having all three greatly increases the dangers. Early detection of females at risk from the triad and appropriate intervention is of the utmost importance.

It is crucial to recognize that menstrual dysfunction is not a normal or necessary consequence of training, but it is a clear sign that health is being compromised. To avoid irreversible skeletal damage, reproductive disorders must be promptly referred to an appropriately qualified medical expert for treatment. Special considerations regarding female athletes are also discussed in chapter 9.

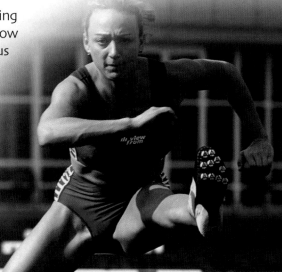

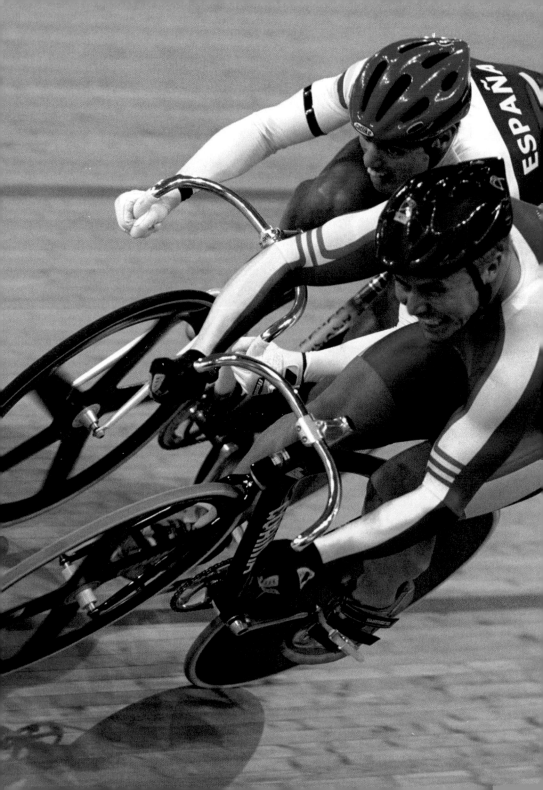

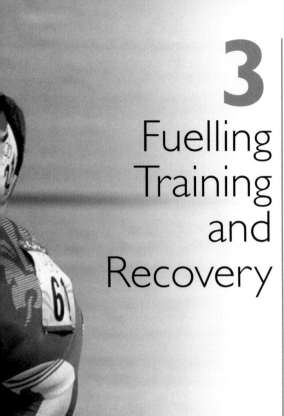

3

Fuelling Training and Recovery

≈ **Carbohydrate is the most important energy fuel**

≈ **Carbohydrate foods should be the main focus of the training diet**

≈ **Body's stores of carbohydrate are limited so need to be restocked between training sessions**

≈ **To sustain training and train again athletes must recover**

≈ **Plan and practise fuelling and recovery strategies during training**

Life in the world of sport revolves around training. However, to be able to train again, as well as strive for performance improvements, be it skill, power, strength, speed or endurance, we need to recover between one training session and the next. So why is there such a huge emphasis on carbohydrates? Well, no matter what type of exercise you do, your body will always use some carbohydrate for energy. But, the body's stores are limited and so need to be restocked in time for the next workout.

The key aspect of the daily diet during training is to ensure that it supplies the body with enough - and the right sort - of energy to fuel training as well as helping the body to adapt and perform. Whatever we're doing, our bodies require energy. But when we train, we need to be able to draw on more of it - faster. Carbohydrate, protein and fat are the three main energy fuels for exercise. However, the preferred energy fuel for the muscles is glucose, especially as exercise intensity increases. Glucose is formed from the breakdown of carbohydrates and is stored as glycogen in the muscles and liver.

However, carbohydrate stores within the body are relatively small and so need to be topped-up daily or even more frequently. If you don't restock your glycogen stores sufficiently, you will run out of fuel after only a few days of training or you will find that you feel fatigued. Therefore it's important to eat enough carbohydrates to not only fuel training, but also to optimize recovery of glycogen stores between training sessions.

General Carbohydrate Recommendations

Just how much carbohydrate you need depends on your level of training - the more glucose you use the more carbohydrate you need to eat to replenish your stores. General daily carbohydrate targets can be provided in terms of body size and training level. Giving carbohydrate targets - and other nutrients like protein - in terms of grams per kg body weight is likely to be more closely related to the muscles' absolute need for fuel than would a guideline in terms of percentage contribution of total energy intake. See Table 1 to work out the amount of carbohydrate - expressed in grams per day for every kilogram you weigh (g/kg/d) - your training programme requires.

Table 1. Carbohydrate recommendations for training

Training level	Carbohydrate g/kg/d
Regular levels of activity (3-5 hrs/week)	4 - 5
Moderate duration/low intensity training (1-2 hrs day)	5 - 7
Moderate to heavy endurance training (2-4+ hrs/day)	7 - 12
Extreme exercise programme (4-6+ hrs/day)	10 - 12

The more intense your training programme, the more carbohydrates you need to eat to ensure successful refuelling and restocking of glycogen stores from day to day - whether it's recovering from daily training sessions or multiple workouts in one day. Planning dietary strategies to meet these targets will be particularly important for athletes whose high training levels are likely to challenge or even exceed the body's normal carbohydrate stores.

If you take these recommendations literally, then you'll see in Table 2 (overleaf), that it produces quite a wide range of daily carbohydrate needs for people of the same body weight, but with different levels of training. In essence, daily carbohydrate requirements may be lower for athletes whose training programmes do not challenge daily glycogen stores, but may be higher for some individuals or some situations. So, it's essential that you're realistic as to how hard and how long you're training on a daily basis - time spent getting changed doesn't count!

As always, it's important to bear in mind that these are simply recommendations from what science has discovered. Tailoring them to suit your individual energy and training needs is down to you. During training take yourself through a trial and error process to fine-tune your actual carbohydrate needs, by taking into account feedback from your energy levels and training performance.

Carbohydrate and Food

Carbohydrates are simply all the sugars and starches in the diet. However, it is important to choose nutrient-rich carbohydrate foods and to add other foods to recovery meals and snacks to provide a good source of protein and other nutrients. The bulk of your carbohydrate intake should come from cereal and starchy sources, the main ones being breads, potatoes, rice, pasta and breakfast cereals, plus the less common starchy vegetables such as sweet potatoes and plantains, as well as peas, beans and lentils. The remainder can come from more sugary sources such as sugar, fruit and juices.

Table 2. Range of carbohydrate needs (g/d)

Training level	Athlete's body weight in kg			
	40	50	60	70
Moderate duration and low intensity	200-280	250-350	300-420	350–490
Moderate to heavy endurance	280-480	350-600	420-720	490-840
Extreme exercise programme	400-480	500–600	600-720	700–840

As most carbohydrate foods, for example potatoes or sugars, are eventually broken down into glucose, one type is not intrinsically better than the other. And if your training levels are high you need to eat a lot of carbohydrates, and, quite frankly, there is only so much bread and pasta you can eat, so this is where sugary snacks and drinks have a useful role to play.

Thanks to food labelling, the majority of packaged foods will tell you how many grams of carbohydrate per 100g - and often per portion - that food contains. Plus, see Table 3 to discover roughly the amount of carbohydrate you are getting from everyday foods and snacks. You can also check your own intake by using the food record and food charts in fuelling fitness extras.

Table 4 (overleaf) gives some one day examples of how to meet carbohydrate needs for three individuals with different activity levels. Very similar foods have been used throughout the three examples to illustrate what happens to foods and quantities in different circumstances.

80	90	100	110	120	130
400-560	450-630	500-700	550-770	600-840	650-910
560-960	630-1080	700-1200	770–1320	840-1440	910-1560
800-960	900-1080	1000-1200	1100-1320	1200–1440	1300-1560

If you are training frequently, then your daily carbohydrate requirement will be high and so you will probably need to eat frequent snacks and meals to achieve this. Therefore, you must remember to look after your teeth by brushing twice a day with a fluoride toothpaste and visiting the dentist regularly.

Table 3. Carbohydrate content of everyday foods

Medium portion of food	Carbohydrate (g)
Baked potato, pasta or rice	60
Bagel, flapjack or slice of fruit cake	40
1 large banana or 50g raisins	35
2 slices of bread, 2 crumpets, or 1 bread roll	30
Muesli, cornflakes, 2 Weetabix or cereal bar	30
50g chocolate, 10 jelly beans or 3 Jaffa cakes	30
500ml sports drink or squash	30
Baked beans (135g) or sweetcorn (100g)	20
200ml orange or apple juice	20
Apple, pear, orange or 2 kiwi fruit	15
2 tsp honey or jam or 150g low-fat yoghurt	15

Table 4(i). Example of carbohydrate per day

A 50kg female undertaking regular activity would need to eat foods containing 200-250g of carbohydrate per day. For example:

Breakfast	
30g cereal with 100ml semi-skimmed milk	30
200ml orange juice	20
Snack	
Medium piece of fruit e.g. pear, orange, apple	15
Lunch	
2 slices bread	30
Banana (large)	35
Evening meal	
Pasta (200g cooked weight)	65
Broccoli and tomato based pasta sauce	15
Apple (large)	20
Total carbohydrate	230 grams

NOTE: This selection is not designed to be a complete and balanced diet. It is meant simply to demonstrate the quantities of food providing sufficient carbohydrate. Only foods containing carbohydrate are listed. Carbohydrate values are rounded to the nearest 5 grams.

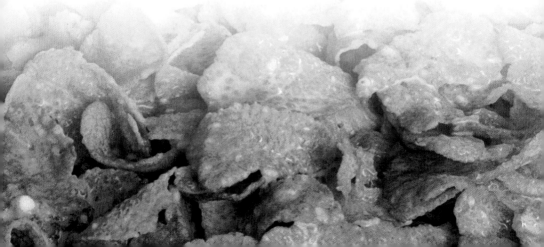

Table 4(ii). Example of carbohydrate per day

A 70kg endurance athlete training 1-2 hours a day would need to eat foods containing 350-490g of carbohydrate per day. For example:

Breakfast	
60g cereal with 200ml semi-skimmed milk	60
2 slices of bread and 2 teaspoons of jam	45
200ml orange juice	20
Post training	
Scone and a low fat fruit yoghurt	35
Medium piece of fruit e.g. pear, orange, apple	15
500ml isotonic sports drink	30
Lunch	
4 slices bread	60
Banana (large)	35
Evening meal	
Pasta (300g cooked weight)	100
Broccoli and tomato based pasta sauce	20
Apple (large)	20
Total carbohydrate	440 grams

NOTE: This selection is not designed to be a complete and balanced diet. It is meant simply to demonstrate the quantities of food providing sufficient carbohydrate. Only foods containing carbohydrate are listed. Carbohydrate values are rounded to the nearest 5 grams.

Table 4(iii). Example of carbohydrate per day

A 90kg power athlete training 2-4 hours a day would need to eat foods containing 630-1080g of carbohydrate per day. For example:

Breakfast	
65g cereal with 568ml (pint) milk	100
4 slices of bread and 4 teaspoons of jam	90
400ml orange juice	40
Post training 1	
Scone with jam or 2 scotch pancakes, and a yoghurt	45
Medium piece of fruit (e.g. pear, orange, apple)	15
500ml isotonic sports drink	30
Lunch	
6 slices bread or 1 baked potato with 200g baked beans	90
Banana (large) and 250ml flavoured milk	60
Post training 2	
Bagel with honey	50
Banana (large) or 50g raisins	35
500ml isotonic sports drink	30
Evening meal	
Pasta (300g cooked weight)	100
Broccoli and tomato based pasta sauce	20
Apple	15
A tin of rice pudding low fat (425g)	60
500ml squash or diluted juice	30
Supper	
90g cereal with 400ml milk	80
Total carbohydrate	890 grams

NOTE: This selection is not designed to be a complete and balanced diet. It is meant simply to demonstrate the quantities of food providing sufficient carbohydrate. Only foods containing carbohydrate are listed. Carbohydrate values are rounded to the nearest 5 grams.

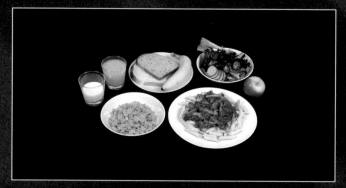

A 50kg female undertaking regular activity would need to eat foods containing 200-250g of carbohydrate per day.

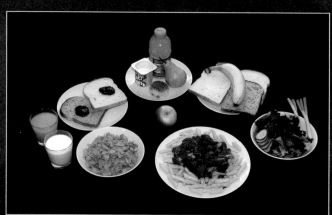

A 70kg endurance athlete training 1-2 hours a day would need to eat foods containing 350-490g of carbohydrate per day.

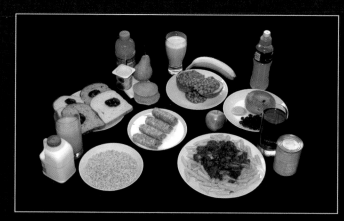

A 90kg power athlete training 2-4 hours a day would need to eat foods containing 630-1080g of carbohydrate per day.

Type of Carbohydrate

The next question to consider is: which type of carbohydrate? Research has shown that a diet high in carbohydrate, obtained either from simple sugars or complex carbohydrates, is equally effective in improving exercise performance. However, perhaps what is more important is how quickly carbohydrate is converted to glucose - and that's where the glycaemic index (GI) comes in.

The GI of a food is a measure of that food's effect on blood glucose levels. It is worked out by comparing the rise in blood glucose after eating a food containing 50g of carbohydrate with the blood glucose rise after eating 50g of a reference food (usually glucose). The larger the rise in blood glucose, the higher the GI (and generally the greater the insulin response). Generally, foods are divided into three categories - high, moderate and low GI. Unfortunately, there is no easy way to tell what the GI of a food is. Some sugars have a high GI (glucose) and others a low GI (fructose). Some complex carbohydrates have a low GI (pasta) whereas others have a higher GI (rice). See Table 5 for the GI category of some everyday foods.

It's important to note that the GI classification is not intended to rank the merits of carbohydrate-rich foods. There are a number of other characteristics of foods, which may be more useful to the athlete - these are often specific to the individual and exercise situation.

Carbohydrate-rich foods with a moderate-high GI provide a fast and readily available source of carbohydrate for glycogen storage and therefore should be the major fuel choice in recovery meals to boost post-exercise refuelling.

It has been suggested that low-GI foods are a good thing to eat before exercise, however in practice there are many other factors that come into play such as comfort, nerves, food preparation etc. This theory assumes that they provide an energy source with minimal insulin response and therefore encourage the body to greater fat burning. However, this theory is not well founded, and it is also irrelevant because insulin secretion is suppressed during exercise. In addition, the rate of glucose supply to the bloodstream from the digestion of low-GI foods is generally not fast enough while exercising.

Table 5. The glycaemic index (GI)

	Rapidly absorbed carbohydrate ⟶ Slower absorbed carbohydrate		
	High GI	**Moderate GI**	**Low GI**
Sugars	Glucose	Sucrose Honey	Fructose Lactose Jam
Fruit	Watermelon Lychees	Banana Pineapple Apricots Paw paw	Peach Apple Pear Orange Grapes Plums
Vegetables	Parsnips Pumpkin Broad beans	Sweetcorn Beetroot	Carrots Peas Baked beans
Breads	French baguette Bagel White, Brown & Wholemeal breads	Pitta bread Muffin (e.g. bran, blueberry) Crumpet	Fruit loaf Rye bread Granary bread
Cereals	Weetabix Cornflakes Bran Flakes Coco Pops	Frosties Porridge	Muesli All-Bran
Starches	Baked potato Mashed potato	White, Brown & Basmati rice Cous cous Sweet potato Boiled & New potato	Pasta Lentils Yam
Snacks	Dried dates Pretzels Jelly beans Popcorn Rice cakes	Raisins Sultanas Mars bar	Dried apricots Peanuts Cashew nuts Fruit & Sponge cake Chocolate
Drinks	Sports drinks	Soft drinks Squash	Milk & Yoghurt Apple juice Orange juice

NOTE: Foods have been categorized according to their average GI value. Several foods cross two categories, e.g. most fruit GI values are between 40-60. GI differs between brands and also country of origin. For example, some muesli and some rye bread will be moderate GI.

One of the problems with low GI carbohydrate foods may be down to the presence of dietary fibre, resulting in a considerable proportion of indigestible carbohydrate. This means that although the food in theory supplies a certain amount of carbohydrate, some is malabsorbed, and is therefore not available to the muscles for refuelling. So, if for an individual, low GI carbohydrate foods are a more normal dietary pattern, it may simply mean that more carbohydrates need to be eaten in order to take account of the indigestible proportion and thereby ensure enough carbohydrates are provided for refuelling the muscles.

Timing of Carbohydrate

The total amount of carbohydrate an athlete consumes is the most important dietary factor in terms of restocking glycogen stores. Other dietary strategies such as timing of intake, type of carbohydrate, or addition of other nutrients, may either directly enhance glycogen recovery or improve the practical aspects of achieving carbohydrate intake targets. As always it's important to try out any new fuelling strategies during training, particularly ingestion of carbohydrates before

and during exercise, to find out what works for your individual requirements. Try different snacks to find which ones suit you best. See Table 7 for some suggestions.

Before training
Carbohydrate requirements in the hours and minutes before exercise - for both training and competition - are covered in more detail in the section on optimizing competition performance. Although you need to allow 2-4 hours after a large meal before exercising, a high carbohydrate snack 30-60 minutes before exercise can be beneficial for some individuals, providing enough carbohydrate is eaten. If pre-exercise carbohydrate is the only means of increasing carbohydrate availability during exercise, then it is important that a reasonable amount - perhaps as much as 100g - is eaten. In general it is best to opt for a high GI carbohydrate, although if carbohydrate is going to be eaten during prolonged exercise the GI of the pre-exercise snack is not so important. However, it is probably advisable to avoid the more bulky (fibre-rich) carbohydrates, as these can cause abdominal discomfort.

During training
In terms of proven performance benefits there are no nutrients that match water and/or

carbohydrate. When carbohydrates are eaten immediately before exercise or during rest periods in prolonged exercise (lasting more than 40 minutes) it is sometimes beneficial to continue to ingest 30-60g carbohydrate per hour throughout exercise to help maintain the flow of glucose.

During exercise that lasts for longer than an hour and which brings about fatigue, it is advisable to consume 30-60g per hour of rapidly absorbed carbohydrate (moderate-high GI), because it generally improves performance. This intake is best achieved by taking feedings every 10-30min, depending on what's allowed in competition for the event, and should be continued throughout the event so that it provides a steady flow of glucose into the blood-stream. The carbohydrate can be in the form of glucose, sucrose, maltodextrins or some high GI starches. Fructose intake should however be limited to amounts that do not cause abdominal discomfort. One of the best ways to achieve this is by drinking a sports drink, which allows carbohydrate and fluid needs to be met (see section on liquids). For example, a carbohydrate intake rate of 30-60g per hour can be met by

drinking 600-1200ml per hour of a sports drink containing 4-8% carbohydrates (4-8g/ 100ml). The higher the carbohydrate content, the less you need to drink.

When exercise does not cause fatigue and is also completed in less than an hour, it is up to individual preference whether to: intake nothing; intake water; or intake water and carbohydrate with or without salt. Furthermore, there seems to be no added benefit - performance or cost - from ingesting other substances, such as glycerol and amino acids, during exercise.

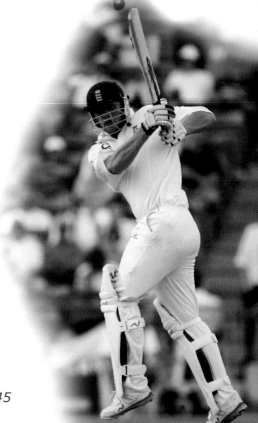

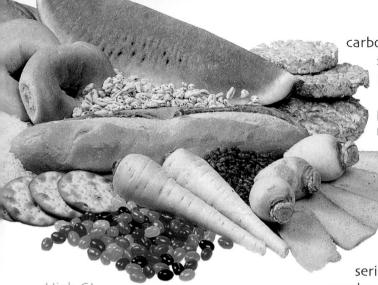

High GI
carbohydrates

carbohydrate intake should start as soon as is practically possible. This means it may be more useful and comfortable to meet the initial carbohydrate target by a series of small snacks - liquids and/or solids - as opposed to large meals. There are plenty of portable high carbohydrate snacks to choose from - see Table 7 for some suggestions.

After training

Recovery is without doubt the most important aspect of training. To sustain training and train again - sometimes more than once in a day - athletes must recover. Nutritional strategies that can optimize recovery are therefore of the utmost importance. Apart from total carbohydrate intake, timing is also key for recovery, because the highest rates of muscle glycogen storage occur in the first few hours after exercise.

It is particularly important that recovery time is used well when there is only a short time - less than 8 hours - between training sessions. In this situation,

Therefore, in the immediate recovery phase - within the first four hours after exercise - it is recommended that around 1-1.2g of carbohydrate per kg of body weight is eaten each hour - see Table 6. Depending on what is practical and comfortable, this can either be met through a single meal or a series of frequent snacks.

Eating some carbohydrate foods immediately after strenuous exercise will not only help the muscle start effective recovery, but also takes advantage of the enhanced rate of glycogen storage at this time.

46

Table 6.
Immediate carbohydrate
needs after exercise (0-4 hrs)

Body weight (kg)	Carbohydrate needs (g/hr)
40	40 - 48
50	50 - 60
60	60 - 72
70	70 - 84
80	80 - 96
90	90 - 108
100	100 - 120
110	110 - 132
120	120 - 144
130	130 - 156

In general, it seems that there is a two hour 'window of opportunity' when glycogen storage rates are best. Then again, effective glycogen storage doesn't happen until carbohydrate is eaten - so storage when carbohydrate is eaten versus no storage when it's not!

When there is a longer recovery period, such as 24 hours between daily training sessions, then the pattern and timing of eating carbohydrate-rich meals and snacks is not so critical, providing the day's carbohydrate target is met. Again preference is down to individual choice, but in terms of restocking glycogen stores, it doesn't matter whether the carbohydrate is consumed as liquid-form or solid foods, or as meals versus frequent snacks.

Lower GI carbohydrates

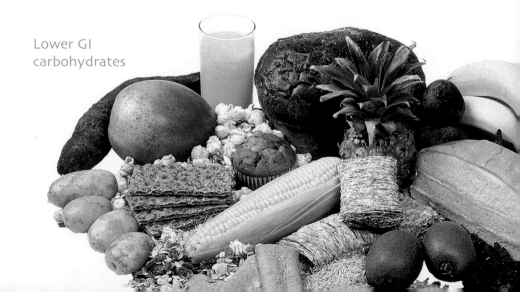

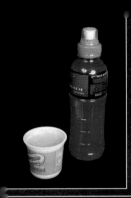

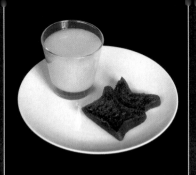

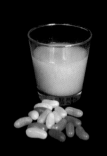

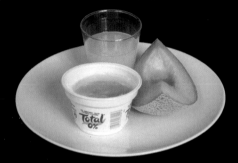

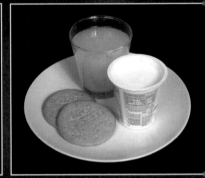

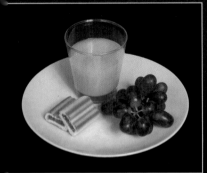

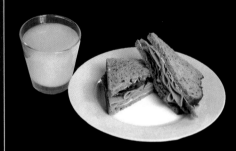

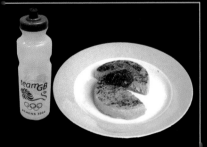

Table 7.
Snacks providing
50g (approx)
carbohydrate

Table 7: Snacks providing 50g (approx) carbohydrate

135g baked beans plus 2 medium slices toast

500ml isotonic sports drink and pot of low-fat custard

200ml orange juice and 2 slices currant bread

30g corn flakes, 1 large kiwi and 200ml low-fat milk

250ml hot chocolate and a wholemeal scone

35g jelly sweets and 150ml glass orange juice

150ml carrot juice, 3 rye crisp breads (cottage cheese to taste) plus 100g fresh pineapple and a small apple

2 medium slices toast, 2 teaspoons jam and 200ml skimmed/ semi-skimmed milk

100g melon, 2 teaspoons honey, 150g pot low-fat plain yoghurt and 150ml apple juice

100g grapes, 2 fig rolls and 150ml orange juice

Lean ham and salad sandwich (2 slices brown bread) and 200ml glass apple juice

175g baked potato (with filling e.g. salad and prawns)

120g sorbet and 200ml orange juice

200g drinking yoghurt and a fruit scone

150g pot low-fat plain yoghurt, 2 digestive biscuits and 200ml apple juice

1 crumpet and a teaspoon of jam plus 500ml isotonic sports drink

250g home-made fruit salad (with equal proportions of banana, orange, apple, pear and grapes) plus 150g low-fat plain yoghurt

1 toasted currant bun plus 200ml pineapple juice

Prawn and salad sandwich on 2 slices of light rye bread, plus 2 small tangerines and 200ml flavoured low-fat milk

Other Nutrients and Recovery

Before considering other nutrients it's important to stress that above all the diet must supply adequate energy intake for optimal glycogen recovery. Restrained eating practices of some athletes, particularly females, and periods of energy restriction make it difficult to meet carbohydrate requirements and to optimize glycogen storage from a low energy intake.

Fluid and salt
Replacement of sweat losses is also an essential part of the recovery process and is discussed in more detail in the section on liquids. Both water and salts lost in sweat need to be replaced. The aim is to drink about 1.2-1.5 litres of fluid for each kg of body weight lost during training. Sodium (salt) can be replaced either via drinks that contain sodium, such as sports drinks, or from food.

Protein
Protein is another nutrient that has received a lot of attention in terms of recovery. The section on protein covers this area in more detail. In general, it seems that when protein is added to carbohydrate during recovery there is more glycogen storage.

However, whether the increase in glycogen storage is simply due to the additional energy from protein or the protein per se, is not known with any certainty. However, in practical terms, when energy intake levels and food availability make it difficult to consume adequate amounts of carbohydrate then the addition of protein to post-exercise meals and snacks may enhance overall glycogen recovery. Besides, dietary protein itself is a useful part of the recovery process, particularly in terms of building and repairing muscles.

Fat
Since the body's fat stores are relatively large, even in very lean athletes, it is generally not necessary to replace fat used as fuel in exercise as it doesn't affect performance. Recently, there has been increased interest in the utilization of IMTG (intramuscular triacylglycerol) fat stores during prolonged moderate-intensity exercise and their replacement during recovery. IMTGs provide a potentially important energy source for the working muscle, but whether exercise performance is affected if they are restocked is currently unresolved. Of course, higher dietary fat intakes will restock IMTG stores quicker than lower fat intakes, but this may

compromise the restocking of glycogen stores and so impair exercise performance. For that reason, it is probably best to concentrate on carbohydrate intake in the initial 6-8 hours of recovery and then rely on regular meals to provide the fat in the diet.

The consumption of excessively large amounts of protein and fat is discouraged as it may displace carbohydrate foods within the total energy requirements of the diet and as a result indirectly interfere with glycogen storage. Consuming excessive amounts of alcohol is also discouraged during the recovery process as it may have an indirect effect on glycogen storage by interfering with the ability, or interest, to follow guidelines for post-exercise eating. Therefore, guidelines for sensible drinking should be followed at all times, and especially in the period after exercise.

Feeling Fatigued?

Runners call it 'hitting the wall', cyclists call it 'bonking' - but what is fatigue and why does it happen? You become sluggish, reaction time slows down, co-ordination and balance start to go, concentration dwindles and you feel light-headed - these are all signs of fatigue.

The main cause of fatigue is due to running out of those vital glucose stores (glycogen) in the muscles - although dehydration alone can also result in fatigue. Therefore, if you want to exercise longer and harder, you need to start each training session with a full tank of glucose - so make sure you thoroughly restock those glycogen stores after training.

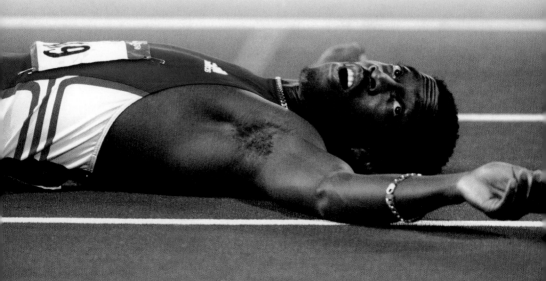

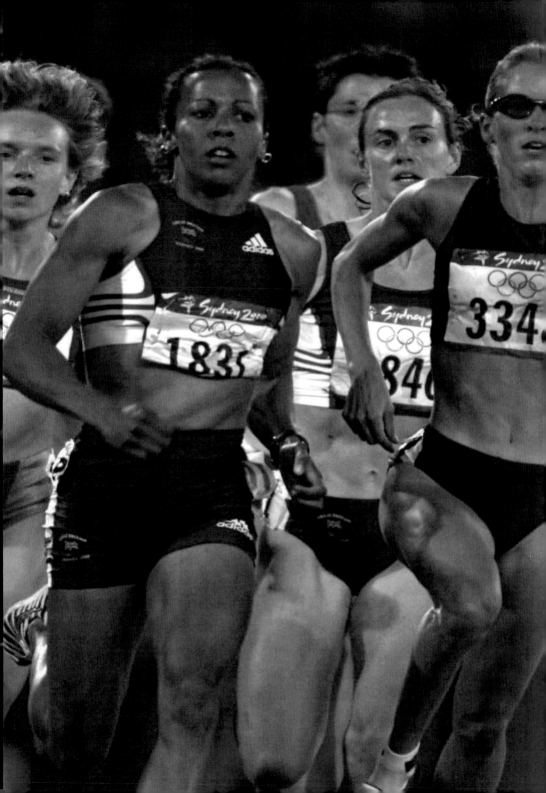

4

The Protein Question

≈ **Protein is required for building and repairing muscle**

≈ **Providing energy needs are met, a varied diet is likely to supply more than enough protein**

≈ **Most athletes do not need to eat extra protein**

≈ **Well chosen vegetarian and vegan diets can meet protein needs**

≈ **Type and timing of eating protein-rich foods may be important**

≈ **Protein and amino acid supplements are not necessary**

Does heavy training require more protein? This seemingly simple question has been hotly debated for years and remains one of the most controversial issues in sports nutrition today. The simple answer is probably no, but of course that depends on what we mean by extra!

Protein has been held in high regard in the competitive arena for longer than most of us can remember - at least as far back as the ancient Olympians. Sure, protein plays an important role in the response to exercise, and in particular, it is needed for building new tissue - including muscle - and repairing the old. But that doesn't necessarily mean that strenuous training, be it strength, speed or endurance work, merits the need for extra protein. In fact, most athletes will find that their protein intakes are high enough because of the extra food they are eating to meet the energy needs of their sport.

With a huge array of sports, and even varying body types for different positions within a single sport, generalization is always tricky. So leaving *requirements* aside for a moment, let's first look at what the *recommendations* are for protein.

General Protein Recommendations

In theory, those following a tough endurance or resistance training exercise programme may need to increase their dietary protein intake above the level that is generally recommended for a healthy, but sedentary, person. The average daily protein recommendations - expressed in grams per day for every kilogram you weigh (g/kg/d) - are summarized in Table 1.

In the UK, the recommended dietary protein intake for people who are sedentary or have low levels of activity, is equivalent to 0.75g per kg of body weight.

Table 1. Daily protein recommendations

Activity level	Protein g/kg/d
Sedentary to low levels of activity	0.75
Regular activity (more than 1 hour per day)	1.0- 1.2
Endurance athletes	1.2- 1.4
Strength or speed athletes	1.2- 1.7

This translates to a 60kg person needing 45g (60 x 0.75) of protein per day. For people who are regularly exercising - more than an hour each day - the recommendation for protein is slightly increased to 1.0 – 1.2g of protein per kg of body weight per day - that's 60 – 72g of protein a day for a person weighing 60kg. However, despite the slight increase in protein requirement, it is still well within - and probably less - than the amount that is typically consumed in Western societies. So there is no need to focus on eating more!

Some, but not all, sports scientists recommend a further increase for athletes in the order of 1.2 - 1.4g/kg/d for endurance athletes and 1.2 - 1.7g/kg/d for strength or speed athletes.

If you take these recommendations literally, then you'll see in Table 2 (overleaf), that they produce quite a wide range of daily protein needs for people of the same body weight, but with different emphases in their training programme.

However, for many sports it is not always possible to simply divide them into strength or endurance categories. So again generalized blanket recommendations are not very helpful. Instead, a more sports, and sometimes also position, specific functional recommendation is required. Other variables also need to be considered, such as: stage of training (starting-out versus established); goals of training and competition; importance and intake of other nutrients (carbohydrates in particular); and perhaps body weight control.

If you take a high protein diet you adapt to this diet and need to continue to consume a high protein intake. But this is not necessary for performance and offers no advantage.

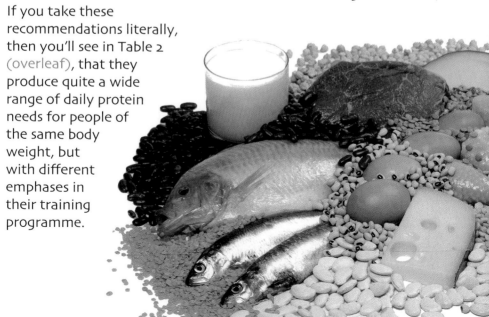

Protein Requirements versus Recommendations

The issue as to whether or not strenuous physical training requires extra protein is more a scientific debate than a practical one. There are pros and cons on both sides of the argument. Contrastingly, there is also evidence to suggest that exercise may actually decrease protein needs due to an increased efficiency of protein utilization.

Providing energy needs are met, it also seems that lean body mass can be maintained within a wide range of protein intakes. Of course, this may not be the goal of athletes who are trying to increase muscle mass. And, what's more, research shows us that most athletes are already habitually eating more than 1.2 - 1.7g/kg/d - the highest suggested range - and that's even without using protein supplements. So 'extra' protein is already being consumed!

In addition, when protein requirements are increased, for example, during heavy endurance training, the amount of overall energy required is also increased. So providing these energy needs are met from a variety of everyday foods, it is likely that protein intake will also be increased - without having to adjust the foods or composition of the diet. It follows through, that if the diet is severely restricted, either in energy intake or dietary variety, then there is a risk that protein needs - and those of other essential nutrients - may not be met.

Table 2. Range of daily protein needs (g/d)

Activity level	Athlete's body weight in kg			
	40	50	60	70
Regular	40-48	50-60	60-72	70-84
Endurance	48-56	60-70	72-84	84-98
Strength & speed	48-68	60-85	72-102	84-119

It's important to note, that experts also state that there is no advantage - either in terms of performance or muscle size - in taking more than 2g of protein per kg of body weight per day (providing carbohydrate needs are met). However, many strength athletes and bodybuilders report consuming protein in excess of 2 - 3g/kg/day. This is often in the belief that excess protein will lead to an increase in muscle mass but, in reality, the extra protein is metabolized and excreted, rather than converted into muscle.

Although such high protein diets are not necessarily harmful, they are expensive, and also carry the risk of displacing other nutritional goals, such as providing adequate fuel for continued training and performance.

In fact, it is entirely feasible that an increase in energy intake is fundamental for increasing muscle mass during training, possibly more so than protein intake. But, it's important to ensure that this tactic fits within the other training and competitive goals and does not lead to an undesirable increase in fat mass.

Protein and Food

In practice, providing enough food is consumed to meet both energy and carbohydrate requirements, then achieving an adequate amount of protein is fairly easy. Table 3 (overleaf) lists some everyday protein-rich foods. You can also check your own intake using the food record and food charts in fuelling fitness extras.

Athlete's body weight in kg					
80	90	100	110	120	130
80-96	90-108	100-120	110-132	120-144	130-156
96-112	108-126	120-140	132-154	144-168	156-182
96-136	108-153	120-170	132-187	144-204	156-221

Table 3. Protein-rich foods

10g Protein is provided by:
30g lean meat or poultry
40g fish
70g soya beans
125g tofu, lentils, kidney beans
Small tin (225g) baked beans
50g nuts or seeds
2 small eggs
330ml cow's milk
400ml soya milk
30g skimmed milk powder
200g yoghurt
40g hard cheese (e.g. cheddar)
110g breakfast cereal
3 slices of bread

Animal sources are richer in protein than vegetable sources and, therefore, a larger quantity of non-animal sources need to be consumed to provide the equivalent amounts of protein. This can be particularly problematic for vegetarian strength and endurance athletes due to the bulk of the fibre-rich vegetables and pulses that they need to eat to meet daily protein needs. In this situation protein intake needs to be monitored and it may be necessary to supplement the diet with a rich source of protein such as milk powder.

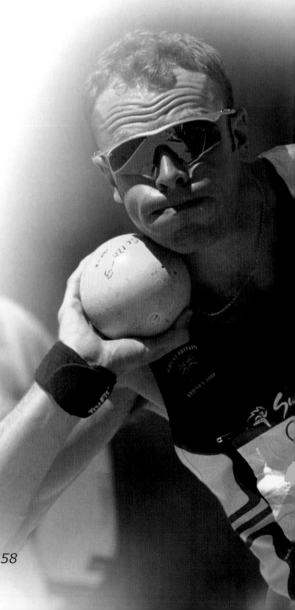

Table 4(i). Example of protein per day

A 50kg person undertaking regular activity would need to eat foods containing 50-60g of protein. For example:

Breakfast	
30g cereal with 100ml milk	5
Lunch	
Quarter a tin tuna in brine (50g)	12
2 slices bread	6
Evening Meal	
50g chicken breast (grilled meat only)	16
Pasta (200g cooked weight)	13
Broccoli and tomato based pasta sauce	6
Apple (large)	1
Total protein	59 grams

NOTE: This selection is not designed to be a complete and balanced diet and it may not contain enough carbohydrate to cover training. It is meant simply to demonstrate the quantities of food providing sufficient protein.   Only foods containing protein have been listed.   Protein values are rounded to the nearest gram.

Table 4 gives some one day examples of how to meet protein needs for three individuals with different activity levels. Very similar foods have been used throughout the three examples to illustrate what happens to foods and quantities in different circumstances.

Table 4(ii). Example of protein per day

A 70kg endurance athlete would need to eat foods containing 84–98g of protein. For example:

Breakfast	
40g cereal with 100ml milk	7
1 slice of bread	3
Post Training	
Scone and a low fat fruit yogurt	9
Lunch	
Half a tin tuna in brine (100g)	24
2 slices of bread	6
Banana (large)	2
Evening Meal	
75g chicken breast (grilled meat only)	24
Pasta (200g cooked weight)	13
Broccoli and tomato based pasta sauce	8
Apple (large)	1
Total protein	97 grams

NOTE: This selection is not designed to be a complete and balanced diet and it may not contain enough carbohydrate to cover training. It is meant simply to demonstrate the quantities of food providing sufficient protein. Only foods containing protein have been listed. Protein values are rounded to the nearest gram.

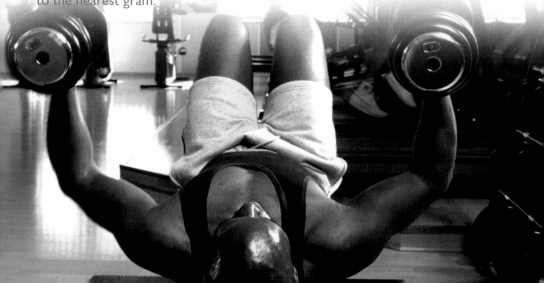

Table 4(iii). Example of protein per day

A 90kg strength athlete would need to eat foods containing 100-153g of protein. For example:

Breakfast	
80g cereal with 200ml milk	13
3 slices of bread	9
Post Training	
Scone and a low fat fruit yogurt	9
Lunch	
Half a tin tuna in brine (100g)	24
4 slices of bread	12
Banana (large)	2
250ml flavoured milk	9
Evening Meal	
100g chicken breast (grilled meat only)	32
Pasta (300g cooked weight)	20
Broccoli and tomato based pasta sauce	8
Apple (large)	1
Supper	
80g cereal with 200ml milk	13
Total protein	152 grams

NOTE: This selection is not designed to be a complete and balanced diet and it may not contain enough carbohydrate to cover training. It is meant simply to demonstrate the quantities of food providing sufficient protein. Only foods containing protein have been listed. Protein values are rounded to the nearest gram.

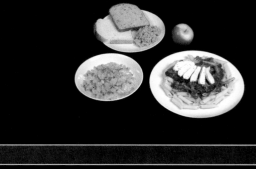

Table 4(i).
A 50kg person undertaking regular activity would need to eat foods containing 50-60g of protein.

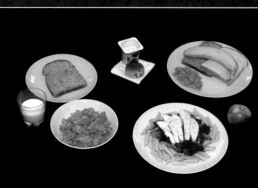

Table 4(ii).
A 70kg endurance athlete would need to eat foods containing 84–98g of protein.

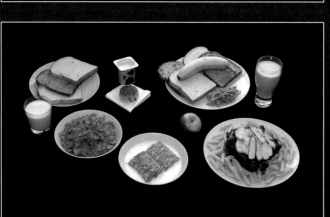

Table 4(iii).
A 90kg strength athlete would need to eat foods containing 108-153g of protein.

Muscle Recovery

Dietary protein intake is needed for the recovery process following training, particularly in terms of the muscles. Research has found that the recovery process for muscle is enhanced when protein is eaten alongside carbohydrate. Although the research is scant, it seems that the 'window of opportunity' is wider for protein recovery than for restocking glycogen (carbohydrate stores), so protein intake is necessary after a training session but perhaps doesn't need to be quite so immediate.

In terms of resistance training, it may also be beneficial to consume small amounts of protein - around 6g - prior to training. Again, it's important to emphasize that although scientific support is limited, it seems to be more beneficial to consume proteins that are richer in essential amino acids than non-essential amino acids. (See back to basics)

However, a great deal more research is necessary before guidelines can be drawn up regarding the amount, type and timing of protein intake - the definitive study is yet to be done, but then again, may never be done! So, the take home message is that after a heavy training session it might be useful to include a little protein in the post-training snack (see Table 3). Remember that most solid foods as well as milk and milkshakes contain some protein.

It's important to remember that during exercise the body relies mainly on muscle glycogen, liver glycogen and fat stores for fuel. Protein is used as muscle fuel if glycogen stores are low. It is therefore essential to ensure that glycogen (carbohydrate) stores are kept well topped up to stop muscle protein being used as fuel. The best way to achieve this is to ensure the diet is rich in carbohydrate, and where necessary eat additional carbohydrate before, during and after exercise.

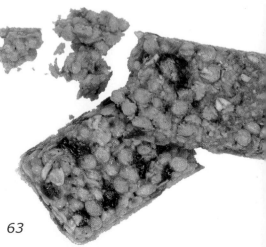

Protein and Amino Acid Supplements

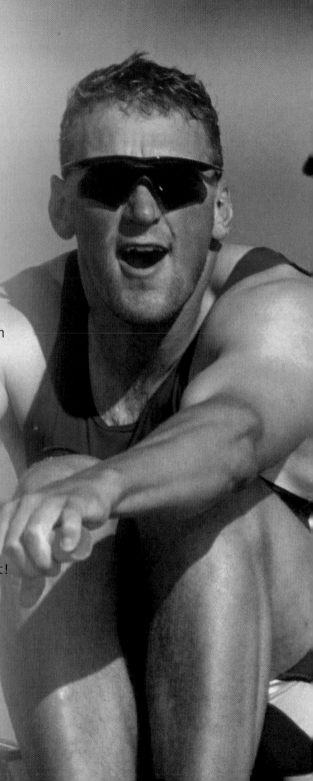

It is simple to meet protein needs from everyday foods. This still holds true when dietary fat intake needs to be controlled. When a period of strict restriction of dietary fat is required it would still be best to carefully select protein foods - and cooking methods - before resorting to using protein supplements. In these situations, it is strongly recommended that advice is sought from a sports nutrition expert, such as a sports dietitian or registered sport and exercise nutritionist.

High-protein diets have been falsely associated with exercise training, due to the mistaken belief that this will lead to greater muscle mass and strength, simply because muscle itself is protein. But, despite the influential power of advertising, a protein supplement will primarily just burn a large hole in your pocket! Nor is there any benefit in taking expensive amino acid supplements. It doesn't matter if excess protein is obtained from food or a supplement it still won't be turned into muscle!

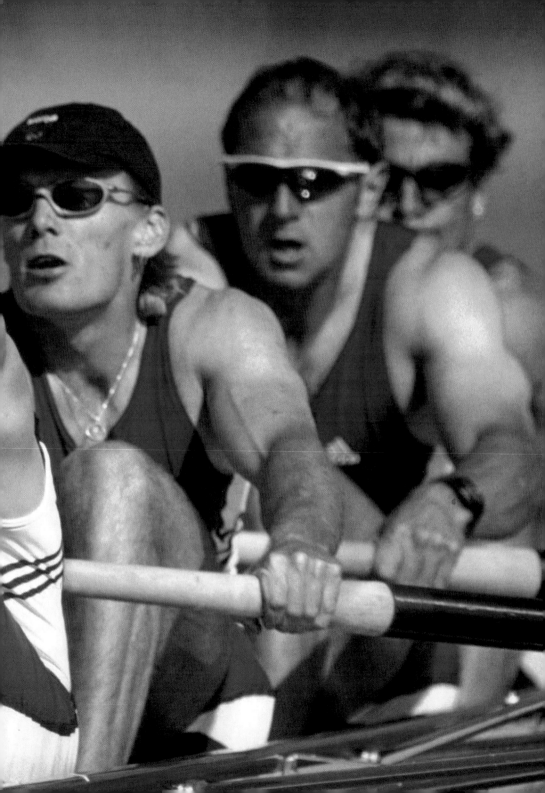

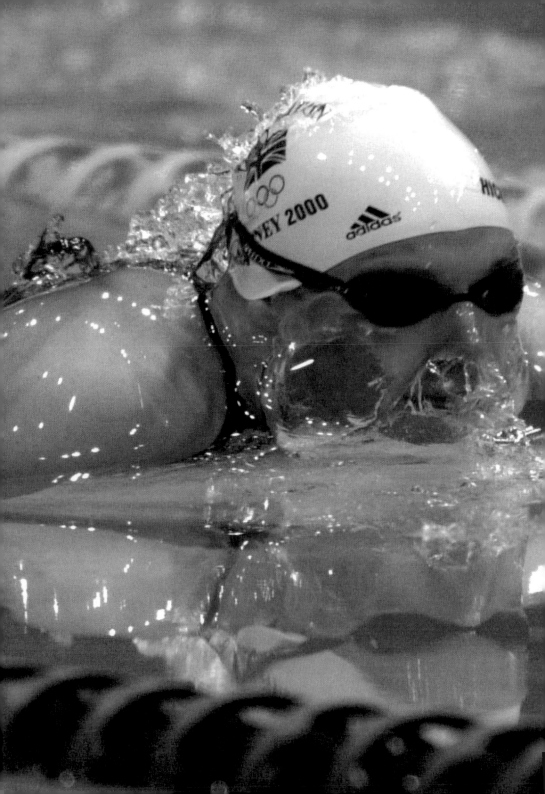

5

Liquid Assets

≈ **Start each training session well hydrated**

≈ **Calculate sweat losses by measuring body weight before and after training sessions to determine how much fluid you need**

≈ **Limit fluid losses to less than 1-2% of body weight**

≈ **Don't drink so much that you actually gain body weight during exercise**

≈ **After exercise aim to drink about 1.2-1.5 litres of fluid for each kg of body weight lost during training and competition**

≈ **Sports drinks provide both carbohydrate and fluid and are useful for intense exercise that lasts longer than about an hour**

≈ **Plan and practise drinking strategies during training sessions**

We all know we should drink plenty of fluids every day to stay hydrated, but how do we know how much is needed to replace the sweat losses during and after exercise? Not enough and exercise performance is compromised, too much and we risk developing hyponatraemia.

When we exercise, our muscles only use about 25 per cent of the energy for work, with the rest released as heat - which is why exercise makes you hot! The main way the body is kept cool is by sweating. Heat from the working muscles is transferred to the blood. The blood flow to the skin is increased, and heat is lost by evaporation - sweating. Sweat comes from the water in the body, so we need to replace this vital fluid to prevent dehydration. If we exercise while dehydrated, our temperature can rise quickly and cause heatstroke, which is potentially fatal.

Replacing fluid lost during exercise is crucial and becomes even more important in hot and humid conditions. If the fluid shortfall is too great then it is likely that exercise performance will be compromised. To effectively restore hydration levels after exercise it is necessary to drink fluid in excess of the sweat losses, and at the same time replace the salts, particularly sodium, that are also lost in sweat.

Optimizing the recovery process is particularly important when there is only a short time between training sessions. It is therefore useful to think of the post-exercise recovery being the pre-exercise preparation. After all, with so much of the focus being on training, it's important

to recover sufficiently so that you're ready to train again, be it in a few hours time or the next day. Along with other aspects of training it's important to tailor your fluid requirements to suit the specific challenges of your sport, paying particular attention to the environmental conditions.

Fluid Requirements

In general, we need about 2-3 litres of fluid a day to be properly hydrated - about half of this normally comes from food and half from drinks. However, it's quite likely that exercise will increase our fluid needs. The more you sweat, the more you need to drink to replace the lost fluid. Some people naturally sweat heavily, but even small sweat losses can cause fatigue, especially in hot weather. Plus, the fitter you are, the more effectively you keep your body cool - so the more you sweat! Training harder, longer or in hot and humid surroundings will also make you sweat more.

During training and competition it's important to limit dehydration by trying to drink at a rate that limits body weight losses. But don't leave it to voluntary fluid intake as you're likely to only replace about half of what you've lost! The best way to estimate how much fluid (sweat) you lose is to weigh yourself before and after at least one hour of exercise under conditions similar to competition or hard practice. It's preferable to weigh yourself naked, or at least in minimal clothing, so as not to include the sweat absorbed within your clothing. For estimating sweat rates, the following points are important:

- Wear the minimum of clothes and rub off any sweat from the body with a towel

- Remove trainers and socks

- Pass urine prior to weighing before exercise

- Weigh yourself as soon as is practical after exercise (within 10 mins) and before passing urine

- Record the amount of fluid you drink during the training session either by weighing the bottle or by marking the bottle

- Remember, the aim is to limit fluid losses - not to lose too much or to gain weight

Each kg of weight loss is equivalent to one litre of fluid loss. However, you will lose more fluid as urine and you will continue to sweat after exercise, so the amount of fluid needed is estimated to be 1.2-1.5 times the fluid lost - so that's 1.2-1.5 litres of fluid for every kg of weight lost. Table 1 gives a couple of examples of how to calculate the fluid loss during exercise and therefore the amount of fluid required to replace sweat losses during recovery.

Table 1. How to calculate the amount of fluid lost

Initial weight	Final weight	Weight difference	Fluid drunk during session	Total fluid loss	Total fluid needed	Extra fluid needed during recovery
a	b	c = a-b	d	Y= c+d	Z = Y x (1.2 or 1.5)	Z-d
70kg	69kg	1kg lost (1000ml lost)	500ml	1000 + 500 = 1500ml	1800 to 2250ml	1300 to 1750ml
72kg	72.5kg	0.5kg gain (500ml gained)	1500ml	1500 - 500 = 1000ml	1200 to 1500ml	None

If you want to work out sweat rate per hour, it's easier to weigh yourself before and after an hour of normal training during which you don't take on fluids - providing the environment is temperate and doing so does not cause you to feel ill. The body weight lost is your sweat loss per hour. So a 1kg body weight loss is 1000ml per hour or 500ml in half an hour. When it's not possible to weigh yourself before and after exercise, another good indicator of fluid loss is to look at the colour of your urine. If it's pale and plentiful, you're well hydrated, but if it's dark and sparse, you probably need more fluid.

If it's not possible to drink enough to prevent some degree of body weight loss during training and competition, then try to limit dehydration levels to no more than about 2% loss of body weight. That's equivalent to 1kg for a person weighing 50kg, 1.5kg for a 75kg person and 2kg for someone who weighs 100kg. However, tolerable losses are smaller in hot and humid conditions and during endurance events. Conversely, it's also important to avoid overcompensating for sweat losses by drinking so much that you actually gain weight during exercise as this can also cause problems.

If you sustain long training sessions, particularly in hot environments, without replacing any fluid, then you will become increasingly dehydrated. This can lead to a rise in body temperature, light-headedness and nausea and, ultimately, you could become fatigued or suffer heatstroke. The best way to prevent this is to start off well hydrated and stay that way!

Drinking Schedule

It is vital that you drink plenty of fluids to avoid compromising your health as well as exercise performance. To succeed, you need to plan your drinking strategies and get into the habit of drinking, so that your body can gradually adapt to the necessary fluid intakes required for your level of training and competition. As with any new sports kit you wouldn't want to try it out during an important competition - the same applies for fluid and fuel strategies! So, simulate competition in training to help you work out your likely fluid needs. Plus, don't leave it to chance, take your beverage choice with you, and keep it with you while you work out or compete.

It's best that you start each training session, race or match fully hydrated. It is often useful to drink in the hours before exercise to ensure normal hydration levels and so correct any possible fluid shortages. However, over-hydrating - for example using glycerol - prior to exercise does not appear to have any meaningful advantage and besides, in healthy individuals the kidneys will excrete the excess fluid before exercise begins. Table 2 (overleaf) gives a summary of how to approach hydration before, during and after exercise. It's important to bear in mind that these are simply recommendations from what the science has discovered. Tailoring them to suit your individual needs and preferences is down to you.

After exercise you need to replace not only water lost as sweat but also salt losses. One of the main factors influencing fluid needs during and after exercise is the volume of fluid lost. So, back to length and type of exercise and likely sweat rates to know the volume of fluid needed. It is unlikely that you will drink too much water during exercise - not drinking enough is usually the problem - but this still doesn't mean you should drink so much that you gain weight. The main time that drinking too much plain water could cause a problem is if you're sweating very heavily for a prolonged period of time, as this could lead to hyponatraemia - low blood sodium levels.

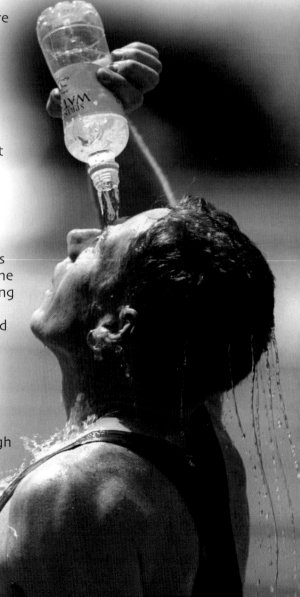

Table 2. Hydration and exercise

Before exercise

- Always start every exercise session well hydrated

- Drinking 400-600ml of water, sports drinks or other fluids in the 2 hours before exercise will help hydrate the body

- Before long or endurance events, drinking 300-500ml of fluid in the 10-15 minutes prior to the start may help the body to absorb fluid more effectively

During exercise

- Aim to drink enough to limit fluid lost as sweat

- Try not to lose more than 1-2%, especially in endurance events in the heat

- This is calculated by taking body weight before and after exercise (see Table 1)

- Every athlete should develop their own strategy for drinking during sport where it is necessary

- For exercise that lasts over an hour, a guide might be to aim to drink 150-250ml every 15 minutes throughout exercise to offset fluid losses

- Drinking smaller volumes more frequently minimizes stomach discomfort

- Those undertaking prolonged exercise should be careful about the amount of fluid drunk. For example - running the average marathon will need 2-4 litres of fluid - that's about 250ml every 2 miles. Those taking a long time to complete an event should not drink large amounts frequently, so as to avoid over-hydration

- Don't drink so much that you actually gain weight during exercise

After exercise

- How much fluid you need depends on how much you have lost

- Drink 1.2-1.5 litres of fluid for every kg of weight lost during exercise

Hyponatraemia

In milder forms, hyponatraemia causes bloating and nausea, and in more serious cases can lead to headaches, confusion, difficulty in breathing, loss of coordination, unusual fatigue, and even death. However, you do have to drink extreme amounts to get it - hence the guideline of 2-4 litres being adequate for most marathon runners. There are two main reasons why excessive drinking can cause this problem. Firstly, because urine production is decreased during exercise, this limits the body's ability to excrete excess fluids. Secondly, sodium is also lost in sweat making it easier for the body's sodium levels to become diluted.

Women doing endurance workouts like marathon running or long cycle rides can be at particular risk, as they are drinking and working out for a prolonged period. This is partly due to women being smaller than men, which means their body fluids get diluted quicker, and because they also tend to be slower, they sweat less and so don't need to drink as much in the first place.

However, it's important to remember that although dehydration is the primary challenge for the majority of athletes, hyponatraemia should be recognized as a possible threat to those who go overboard in their drinking practices. Therefore, during long periods of exercise or competition - lasting longer than two hours - a sports drink containing sodium can be useful in helping replace the salts lost in sweat.

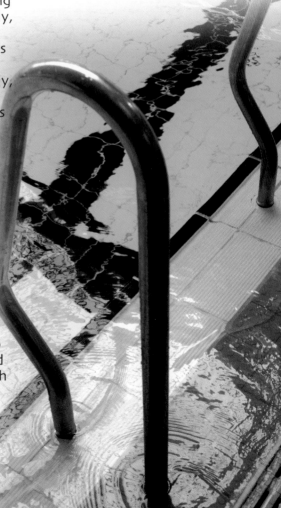

Beverage Choice

The composition of drinks is another key factor to consider in terms of beverage choice during and after exercise. Which fluid you opt for depends on how hard and for how long you are exercising. However, it's important to choose a flavour you like to encourage you to drink more. Table 3 gives a summary of the different types of drinks available for different situations.

Table 3. Beverage choice

Water
When sweat losses are small water is fine. Under these conditions, salt can be obtained from meals and snacks eaten around training.
Hypotonic
These have a lower concentration than blood and so diluted soft drinks and sports drinks containing a small amount (under 4%, i.e. <4g/100ml) of carbohydrate fall into this category.
Hypotonic drinks will generally provide fewer calories per 100ml than isotonic and hypertonic drinks.
Some athletes (e.g. those practising high intensity exercise) find these easier to tolerate and experience less stomach discomfort than when they use isotonic drinks.
Isotonic
Many commercial sports drinks are 'isotonic'. They usually contain 4-8% (4-8g/100ml) carbohydrate and some salt.
They can be useful when exercise is prolonged and can be drunk before, during and after sport.
Sports drinks provide a source of carbohydrate, salt and fluid.
Hypertonic
Contain over 8% (>8g/100ml) carbohydrate and are less quickly absorbed than isotonic and hypotonic drinks.
Useful when energy and carbohydrate needs are high and sweat rates are lower, and also for refuelling after heavy exercise.
Fruit juice, energy drinks and sugary carbonated drinks fall into this category, but they generally don't contain salt and are not ideal to use to hydrate during exercise lasting longer than 1-2 hours.

If you're exercising at a low-to-moderate intensity for less than an hour, then water is great. If you find it difficult to drink large quantities of plain water, try adding some juice or squash, which will also provide you with some carbohydrates to help restock glycogen (carbohydrate) stores.

Beverage choice during exercise
During exercise that lasts for longer than an hour and which elicits fatigue, it is advisable to consume 30-60g per hour of rapidly absorbed carbohydrate, because it generally improves performance. In this instance, a sports drink would be useful.

Sports drinks provide both carbohydrate and fluid simultaneously to help prevent fatigue. Most commercial sports drinks are 4-8% carbohydrate (i.e. they have 4-8g of carbohydrate per 100ml of fluid), making them 'isotonic' - a similar concentration to blood - and, therefore, are quickly absorbed. The carbohydrate can come from sugars (glucose, sucrose, and syrups which contain no more than about 50% fructose), maltodextrins or other rapidly absorbed carbohydrates.

In addition, sports drinks contain sodium to stimulate sugar and water absorption, and replace the sodium lost in sweat. This added sodium is particularly useful if you're exercising for longer than 2 hours or for individuals during any event that stimulates heavy sodium losses - i.e. more than 3-4g of sodium. However, it's difficult to estimate how much sodium you are losing. But, basically, 'salty sweaters' need more sodium. So if you are someone whose sweat is opaque, tastes salty, and leaves white marks on your clothes, then you should probably consider having some extra salt.

Sodium (at moderate concentrations) has the added benefit of encouraging you to drink more. In fact, the drive to drink is present for several hours following exercise (it stops when you eat). However, when your mouth is moistened with fluid, your body automatically signals your brain to stop drinking. This inhibition can happen before the body's fluid levels have been completely restored. This means that even if you don't feel thirsty, you're not necessarily well hydrated, so it's important to keep drinking fluid throughout the day.

Caffeine contained in commonly available beverages can enhance power output during the later stages of endurance performance. This benefit can be obtained with relatively small doses of caffeine - about 1.5mg/kg body weight or approximately 100mg - from commonly consumed drinks such as coffee and cola beverages.

Beverage choice after exercise
The effectiveness of rehydration drinks is a balance between their palatability, promoting intake, and their sodium concentration, promoting fluid retention. Complete restoration of hydration levels can only be achieved if the amount of fluid consumed is greater - 1.2-1.5 times greater - than the amount of fluid lost through sweat. So it's important that you like the taste otherwise you won't drink enough! However, to retain the fluid drunk after exercise it's important that the sodium lost in sweat is also replaced.

Although daily sweat and sodium losses vary widely among individuals and depend on many factors - such as diet, physical fitness, environment and heat acclimatization status - it can be assumed that where sweat losses are high, sodium losses will generally also be high. Therefore, a moderate excess intake of salt would appear to be beneficial for rehydration and

without any detrimental effect on health, providing that fluid intakes are also in excess and kidney function is not impaired.

Consequently, when only liquids are available following exercise it is advisable to consume sports drinks that contain sodium. Alternatively, plain water can be drunk if a source of sodium is available at the same time from (or added to) food. Although other salts are lost in sweat - potassium and magnesium in particular - including these as part of the recovery strategy seems to have no particular benefit over and above sodium.

Although alcohol in moderation is fine, it's certainly not a good idea to drink it just before exercise. You also need to rehydrate properly before drinking alcohol after exercise. Alcohol before exercise not only has a detrimental effect on co-ordination skills and exercise performance, but also increases the risk of injury. Furthermore, alcohol can cause dehydration and slow down recovery from injury.

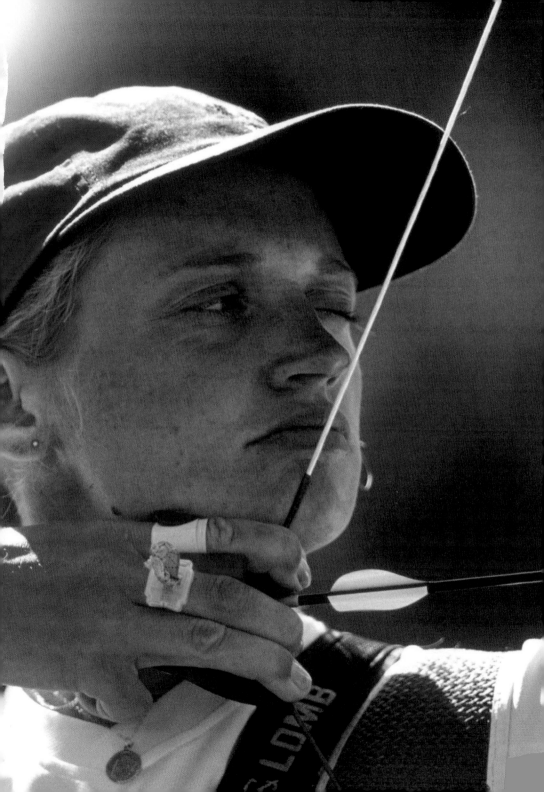

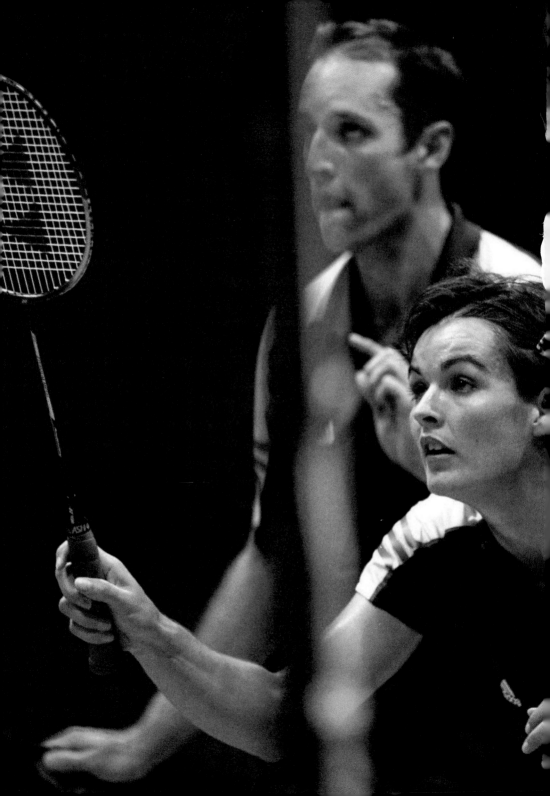

6

Added Extras

≈ Eating a wide variety of foods helps ensure the body's needs for all the micronutrients are met

≈ A wide range of vitamins and minerals are necessary for good health

≈ Athletes do not generally need extra vitamins and minerals

≈ Excessive intake of some micronutrients can be harmful

≈ Micronutrient supplementation does not enhance exercise performance, unless it is needed to correct a pre-existing deficiency

The food we eat provides the nutrients required by the body. However, no single food can provide all the essential nutrients so variety is also key to ensure an adequate supply of micronutrients - vitamins, minerals and antioxidants. If you eat a well balanced diet do you really need extra to keep you on top of your game?

Vitamins and minerals are of great interest in the sports world due to the belief that they will enhance health and improve physical performance. There is no doubt that an adequate supply of a wide-range of vitamins, minerals and trace elements is necessary for good health. Therefore, our dietary intake needs to be sufficient to ensure we meet our body's requirement for all these micronutrients. But, whether exercise increases our requirement is another matter.

The fact is that exercise does not particularly increase the need for vitamins and minerals. Providing you are eating a healthy balanced diet, that is not only adequate in energy but also includes a wide variety of foods, you should have no problem getting all the vitamins and minerals you need.

If you are exercising and not restricting your energy intake, then you will need to eat more food to meet the increased energy demand of your training. More food - providing it's a varied mixture - means you will also be getting more vitamins and minerals.

Although strenuous and prolonged exercise stresses the body, an adequate diet will help ensure good health is maintained. Therefore, even elite athletes, providing the diet is adequate in terms of both quantity and quality, do not usually need extra vitamins and minerals.

Vitamins

Vitamins are a diverse collection of chemicals. They are required in very small quantities - usually only a few micrograms (μg) or milligrams (mg) per day - but are essential for many processes carried out by the body. However, our bodies are unable to make most vitamins and so they need to be supplied in adequate amounts by the diet to prevent deficiency symptoms.

Vitamins are not chemically related, but one of the easiest ways of classifying them relates to their solubility in fat or water. The fat-soluble vitamins are A, D, E and K and the water-soluble vitamins are the B group of vitamins and vitamin C. This classification helps provide some indication of food sources, function and distribution in the body, and potential toxicity - see Table 1.

Table 1. Characteristics of vitamin groups

	Fat-soluble vitamins Vitamins: A, D, E and K	Water-soluble vitamins Vitamins: B group and C
Risk of deficiency	Very low fat diets and conditions where fat absorption is impaired	Diets lacking in variety
Stability in foods	Robust to heat and light	Varies; often unstable when exposed to heat and light
Storage in body	Can be large and long-term	Often small; so frequent regular intakes required
Risk of toxicity	High	Low; as high intakes are usually excreted in urine

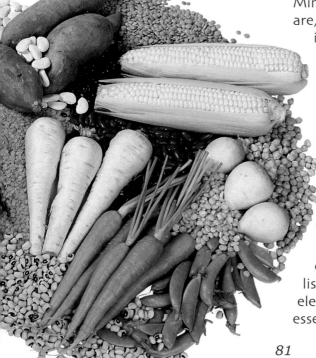

Minerals

Minerals and trace elements are, like vitamins, only required in small quantities, but are nonetheless essential for normal body function. Those required in milligram (mg) quantities (sometimes several hundred milligrams) tend to be referred to as minerals and those required in smaller amounts (micrograms (µg) quantities) are usually called trace elements. Table 2 (overleaf) lists the minerals and trace elements that are known to be essential for humans.

Table 2.
Essential minerals
and trace elements

Minerals	Trace elements
Calcium	Copper
Phosphorus	Chromium
Magnesium	Manganese
Sodium	Molybdenum
Potassium	Selenium
Iron	Iodine
Zinc	

Antioxidants

Muscular exercise results in an increased production of radicals (oxidants) and other forms of reactive oxygen species in the working muscle. Consequently, when a muscle contracts there is oxidative damage, which in-turn could result in muscle fatigue or injury. Muscle cells utilize a network of antioxidants to protect themselves against the risk of oxidative stress and damage. There is some evidence for an adaptive increase in antioxidant status in response to regular exercise, and so this may help protect against further damage.

The common dietary antioxidants are glutathione, vitamin E, vitamin C, lipoic acid, carotenoids, uric acid, bilirubin and ubiquinone. Several minerals also play important, but indirect roles, in providing antioxidant protection in the cells. The minerals and trace elements involved in antioxidant related functions include iron, zinc, copper, manganese and selenium. However, not all antioxidants are created equal and so they may often benefit from working as a network.

Currently, there is limited evidence that dietary antioxidants - above amounts received through the diet - improve exercise performance. It is also not known whether vigorous exercise training requires antioxidants beyond what you would get from a balanced diet with plenty of fruit and vegetables. Consequently, dietary supplementation cannot be recommended at this time. It would therefore be better to adapt the diet to include more dietary sources of antioxidants than experiment with supplements, especially as 'mega-dosing' may actually impair muscular performance. Again too much of a good thing is not necessarily a good thing!

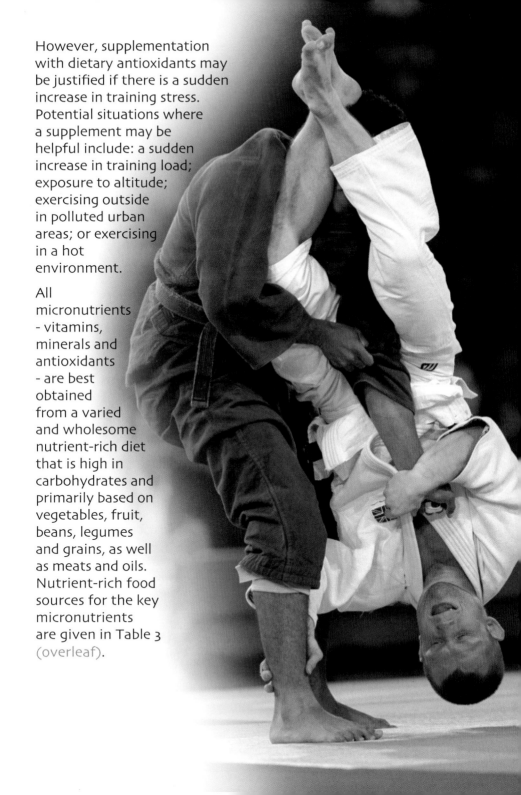

However, supplementation with dietary antioxidants may be justified if there is a sudden increase in training stress. Potential situations where a supplement may be helpful include: a sudden increase in training load; exposure to altitude; exercising outside in polluted urban areas; or exercising in a hot environment.

All micronutrients - vitamins, minerals and antioxidants - are best obtained from a varied and wholesome nutrient-rich diet that is high in carbohydrates and primarily based on vegetables, fruit, beans, legumes and grains, as well as meats and oils. Nutrient-rich food sources for the key micronutrients are given in Table 3 (overleaf).

Table 3(i). Nutrient rich food sources of key vitamins

Micronutrient	What does it do?	Good food sources
Vitamin A (retinol)	Antioxidant function. Cell division & growth, healthy skin & hair. Night vision	Liver & offal, oily fish, eggs, whole milk, cheese, butter, margarine, spinach, broccoli, carrots, red peppers, tomatoes, dark green & orange vegetables
Vitamin B1 (thiamin)	Involved in the release of energy from food. Essential for nervous system	Pork, liver & offal, lean beef, yeast extracts, red kidney beans, potatoes, fortified breakfast cereals, nuts, pulses, whole grains
Vitamin B2 (riboflavin)	Metabolism of carbohydrates & fats	Liver & offal, yeast extracts, green leafy vegetables, dairy products, fortified breakfast cereals & bread
Vitamin B3 (niacin)	Involved in the release of energy from food	Meat & fish, wholegrain & fortified breakfast cereals, yeast extracts, coffee
Vitamin B6 (pyridoxine)	Metabolism of carbohydrate, protein & fats. Important for immune function, formation of red blood cells, maintenance of healthy nervous system	Fortified breakfast cereals, avocado, meat, liver, poultry, fish, eggs, nuts, bananas, soya beans
Folate (folic acid)	Required for cell division & formation of proteins in the body. Extra in pregnancy protects against neural tube defects	Green leafy vegetables, Brussels sprouts, broccoli, spinach, lentils, oranges, fortified breakfast cereals, liver, yeast extracts, wholemeal bread, black eye beans, baked beans

Table 3(i). Nutrient rich food sources of key vitamins continued

Micronutrient	What does it do?	Good food sources
Pantothenic acid	Involved in the release of energy from food	Yeast, offal, peanuts, meat, eggs, green vegetables
Biotin	Involved in metabolism of carbohydrates & fats	Liver & offal, yeast, nuts, pulses, wholegrain cereals, eggs
Vitamin B12 (cyanocobalamin)	Essential for production of red blood cells & to prevent some forms of anaemia. Needed for a healthy nervous system. Used in carbohydrate, protein & fat metabolism	Foods of animal origin e.g. meat, fish, poultry, eggs, dairy & fortified breakfast cereals
Vitamin C (ascorbic acid)	Antioxidant. Healthy skin, gums, blood vessels. Haemoglobin & red blood cell production. Helps absorption of iron from plant foods	Citrus fruits, berries & currants e.g. strawberries & blackcurrants, kiwi, broccoli, green peppers, cabbage, spring greens, potatoes
Vitamin D (cholecalciferol)	Absorption of calcium & regulation of calcium metabolism, healthy bones	Action of sunlight on skin. Oily fish, fortified margarines & breakfast cereals
Vitamin E (tocopherols)	Antioxidant. Promotes normal growth & development	Vegetable oils, wheatgerm, nuts, seeds, margarine, egg yolk, avocado
Vitamin K (phylloquinone)	Essential in formation of certain proteins & normal blood clotting	Green leafy vegetables e.g. spinach, broccoli, green cabbage, Brussels sprouts

Table 3(ii). Nutrient rich food sources of key minerals

Micronutrient	What does it do?	Good food sources
Calcium	Strong bones & teeth. Muscle contraction, blood clotting & transmission of nerve impulses	Milk & dairy products e.g. cheese & yoghurt; fish containing soft bones e.g. sardines & pilchards; fortified white flour products e.g. bread & cereals; dark green leafy vegetables; pulses & seeds
Magnesium	Involved in regulation of energy metabolism. Skeletal development, protein synthesis, muscle contraction & transmission of nerve impulses	Vegetables & potatoes, meats, dairy, pulses, bread & cereals (particularly wholegrain), beer & coffee
Potassium	Works together with sodium to control fluid & electrolyte balance in cells & tissues. Regulates blood pressure	Many plant foods including avocados, nuts, seeds, pulses, potatoes, tomatoes, whole grains & fresh fruit e.g. bananas, oranges. Also meat, fish & dairy
Iron	Antioxidant function. Manufacture of red blood cells. Oxygen transport & utilization. Essential component of wide range of enzymes	Red meat, liver & offal, fortified breakfast cereals, eggs, wholegrain bread & cereals, green leafy vegetables, pulses, dried fruit, nuts & seeds

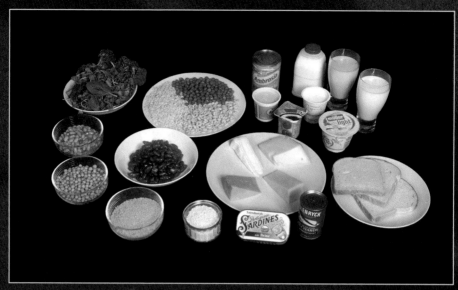

Good sources of calcium

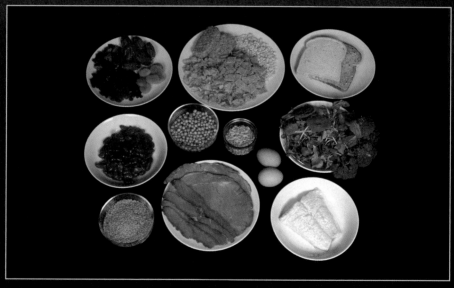

Good sources of iron

Table 3(ii). Nutrient rich food sources of key minerals continued

Micronutrient	What does it do?	Good food sources
Zinc	Antioxidant function. Essential component of wide range of enzymes & vital for normal growth. Assists immune system & helps wound healing	Fish & shellfish, red meat, milk & dairy, poultry & eggs, bread & cereals, green leafy vegetables, pulses
Copper	Antioxidant function. Essential component of wide range of enzymes	Shellfish, liver, nuts, cocoa, meats, cereal products, vegetables & potatoes
Manganese	Antioxidant function. Essential component of wide range of enzymes. Component of bone & cartilage	Tea, bread & cereals (particularly wholegrain), brown rice, pulses, nuts
Selenium	Antioxidant function. Essential component of wide range of enzymes	Fish, meats, fats, vegetables, cereals, lentils, avocados, brazil nuts
Iodine	Works together with thyroid hormones to control heat, protein synthesis & integrity of connective tissue	Seafoods & dried seaweeds, milk & iodized salt

Fruit and Vegetables

For health, it is recommended that we eat at least five portions of fruit and vegetables per day - as they are nutrient-packed and a good source of antioxidants and soluble fibre. It doesn't matter whether they are fresh, frozen, canned, dried, or juiced - although fruit juice can only be counted once even if you drink the whole carton! As always, variety is the key.

However, in the UK, most of us are only managing three portions a day - some individuals don't even manage that. Perhaps this is partly down to not knowing exactly what a portion is. Table 4 demonstrates how the size of the fruit/vegetable affects what constitutes a portion.

Table 4. What is a portion of fruit and vegetables?

	1 large slice of a very large fruit e.g. melon, pineapple
or	1 whole medium fruit e.g. apple, pear, orange
or	2 small fruits e.g. plums, satsumas, kiwi fruit
or	1 cupful of a very small fruit e.g. grapes and berries
or	2-3 tablespoons of fruit salad - fresh, stewed or canned
or	1 tablespoon of dried fruit
or	1 glass (150ml) of fruit or vegetable juice
or	2 tablespoons of vegetables - fresh, frozen or canned
or	1 dessert bowl of salad

Micronutrient Deficiencies

Most active people are highly likely to be meeting their vitamin and mineral requirements by eating a healthy well-balanced diet. Athletes who are undergoing regular strenuous training will need to be eating a high energy diet. Providing that a reasonably varied diet is consumed, it is likely that the high-energy diet will provide micronutrients (vitamins and minerals) in excess of the recommended intake levels for general health. Consequently there is no need to take vitamin and mineral supplements 'just in case'.

There is no sound evidence to suggest that supplementation with vitamins and minerals enhances exercise performance, unless it is needed to correct a pre-existing deficiency. Any marginal deficiency, although it will only have a small impact on body function, may impair exercise performance, especially in individuals where more than one micronutrient is compromised. In theory, it is possible to be deficient in any of the micronutrients, but in practice it is generally uncommon with the exception of calcium and iron.

However, it is not necessary to exceed requirements, and in the case of vitamins, minerals and antioxidants - more does not mean better. Excess intakes of certain micronutrients, particularly the fat-soluble vitamins (A, D, E and K) and iron, can be toxic.

The water-soluble vitamins (the B group and C) are simply passed out in the urine if consumed in excess of requirements.

Table 5.
Diets with a high risk of nutrient deficiencies

Low in energy for weight loss
• especially if followed for a long period
Omitting foods or food groups
• likes/dislikes • vegetarians and vegans
Lacking in a particular type of food
• allergy or intolerance
Erratic and unbalanced
• restricted food intake • disordered eating

Fat-soluble vitamins can accumulate in the body tissues, so if recommended amounts are exceeded over a long period then they may reach toxic levels.

Athletes who have restricted diets may put themselves at risk of inadequate micronutrient intakes. Table 5 gives a list of common dietary situations where there is a higher risk of nutrient deficiencies.

Athletes whose diet puts them at risk of nutrient deficiencies should seek advice from a sports nutrition expert such as a sports dietitian or registered sport and exercise nutritionist before reaching for the supplement jar. When food intake cannot be sufficiently improved, for example when travelling to foreign countries where there is a limited supply of 'safe' food, then a low-dose multi-vitamin and multi-mineral supplement may be necessary. However, single, targeted, nutrient supplements should only be taken under medical supervision for an established nutrient deficiency.

Strict vegetarian diets, although high in carbohydrate and therefore great for providing energy fuel, can without careful planning, lead to micronutrient deficiencies in iron, calcium, iodine, zinc and vitamin B12. Therefore, in this instance, the vegetarian athlete should seek nutritional advice from a sports nutrition expert such as a sports dietitian or registered sport and exercise nutritionist, as to whether supplementation is necessary.

Although some athletes, particularly menstruating females, vegetarians and endurance athletes may have a greater tendency to develop iron deficiency, it is still unwise to routinely take iron supplements. Unexplained fatigue and a fall in sports performance should be fully investigated by a medical professional such as a sports medicine doctor and/or a sports dietitian. Low iron stores can progressively become lower and ultimately lead to problematic iron deficiency. Therefore, athletes who have a high risk of iron deficiency should routinely undergo assessments of their iron status.

Nevertheless, it would still be better to adapt the diet to include more dietary sources of vitamins and minerals than resort to taking a supplement. Simply taking a supplement does not make a bad diet better. Further information can be found in the special considerations sections on female and vegetarian athletes at the end of this book.

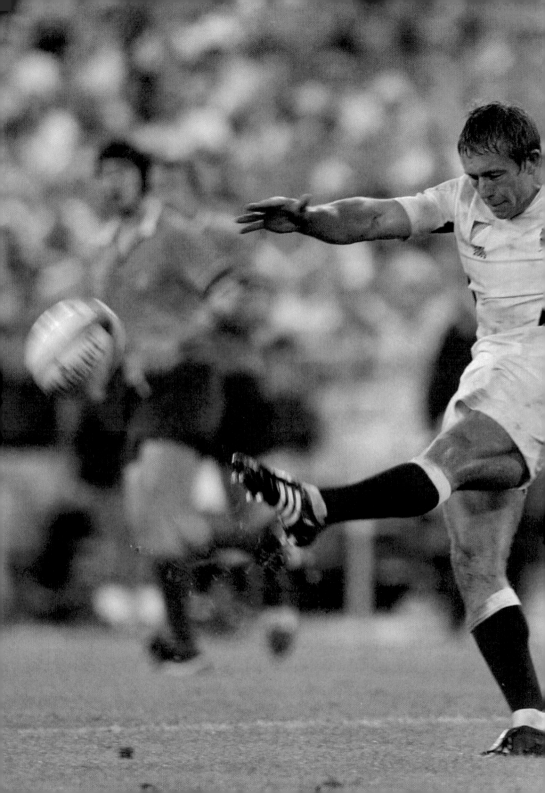

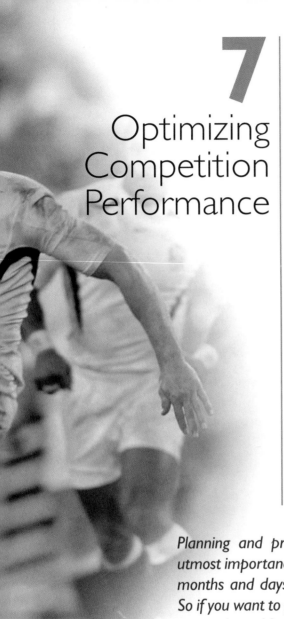

7

Optimizing Competition Performance

≈ **Carbohydrate is the key nutrient for energy, so levels must be optimized prior to competition**

≈ **Water and salt levels also need to be optimized before competing**

≈ **Protein and fat requirements do not increase in the days leading up to competition**

≈ **Carbohydrate loading is particularly beneficial prior to events that last longer than 90 minutes**

≈ **Pre-competition meals should contain sufficient carbohydrate**

≈ **To sustain exercise performance, and compete again, athletes must recover**

≈ **Plan and practise fuelling and hydrating strategies during training - don't try anything new during important competitions**

Planning and preparing for competition is of the utmost importance. After all, it's when all those years, months and days of training will be put to the test. So if you want to perform to your best you need to be at your best. It's not rocket science either - simply get plenty of rest and eat well. Of course defining what, how much, and when to eat is a bit more technical. The focus should be on carbohydrates to ensure your energy tank is full and ready for the off…..

Competition nutrition is all about getting your diet right before, during and in the recovery from the event. And, if you're competing again on the same day then it's even more important that you recover properly before competing again. But of course it's not all about on the day, you also need to prepare in the days leading up to competition, and, in some cases, when competition is scheduled early in the morning there simply aren't hours before the event!

Prior to competition it's essential to make sure all your nutrition 'ducks are in a row'. Otherwise fatigue will set in and your performance will dwindle. Fundamentally, this means you need to have optimally restocked your glycogen (carbohydrate) stores and be adequately hydrated - having also replaced fluid and salt losses - from training. In the final 2-4 days before competition, you will be tapering your training levels and resting more, so your needs for other nutrients, such as protein and fat, will be no different from what is required for a normal moderate level of training. Therefore, the key nutrient to focus on is carbohydrate to ensure that energy stores are optimized prior to competition.

Fuelling up for Competition

It's essential to maximize carbohydrate stores - within both muscle and liver - in the days leading up to competition. If you don't restock your glycogen stores sufficiently following training then you may find you feel fatigued - particularly if your event lasts longer than an hour - and that certainly won't help you perform at your best.

For events that last less than 60-90 minutes muscle glycogen stores can be stocked adequately by resting for 24 hours and eating sufficient carbohydrate - about 7-10g per kg body weight - providing the muscles are not damaged. Therefore, for many athletes, all that's needed to normalize glycogen stores is to schedule a day's rest or light training while continuing to eat a diet rich in carbohydrates. Recommendations for carbohydrate intake levels are covered in more detail in the section on fuelling training and recovery.

Carbohydrate Loading

Athletes who compete intensely for about 90 minutes or more will benefit from carbohydrate loading for a few days before the event. Fortunately, the science has moved on and the diet and exercise regimen for carbohydrate loading is no longer as extreme as it was. Carbohydrate loading is simply about maximizing or supercompensating glycogen stores prior to a competitive event that would otherwise deplete these stores.

Increasing dietary carbohydrate in the week before competition, increases muscle glycogen stores and is associated with enhanced exercise performance in events lasting longer than 90 minutes. This can be achieved by reducing training levels - both intensity and duration - and at the same time eating a large amount of carbohydrate - around 8-10g carbohydrate per kg body weight per day - for 2-3 days. In general, a moderate to hard bout of fatiguing exercise is also performed earlier in the week prior to competition, before the carbohydrate loading phase. It is important to note, that you may find you gain some weight following a carbohydrate loading phase - this is normal. You may also feel heavy in the early stages, but you will feel the benefit later.

Table 1 (overleaf) gives some one day examples of foods providing 8-10g carbohydrate per kg body weight to meet the carbohydrate loading diet needs of three individuals with different body weights. Very similar foods have been used throughout the three examples to illustrate what happens to foods and quantities in different circumstances.

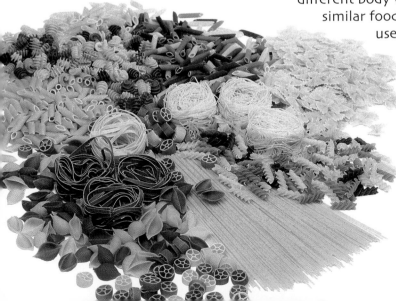

Table 1 (i). Example of carbohydrate loading diet

A 50kg athlete would need to eat foods providing 400-500g of carbohydrate per day. For example:

Breakfast	
30g cereal with 100ml semi-skimmed milk	30
2 slices bread or 2 crumpets with 2 teaspoons of jam	45
150ml orange juice	15
Snack	
Medium piece of fruit e.g. pear, orange, apple	15
500ml sports drink or squash	30
Lunch	
2 slices bread	30
150g low fat fruit yoghurt	10
Banana (large) or 50g raisins	35
Snack	
Bagel with honey or jam	50
Medium piece of fruit e.g. pear, orange, apple	15
500ml sports drink or squash	30
Evening meal	
Pasta (200g cooked weight)	65
Broccoli and tomato sauce	15
Banana (large)	35
Snack	
50g chocolate or cereal bar	30
Total carbohydrate	450 grams

NOTE: This selection is not designed to be a complete and balanced diet. It is meant simply to demonstrate the quantities of food providing sufficient carbohydrate. Only foods containing carbohydrate are listed. Carbohydrate values are rounded to the nearest 5 grams.

Table 1 (ii). Example of carbohydrate loading diet

A 70kg athlete would need to eat foods providing 560-700g of carbohydrate per day. For example:

Breakfast	
60g cereal with 200ml semi-skimmed milk	60
2 slices bread or 2 crumpets with 2 teaspoons of jam	45
150ml orange juice	15
Snack	
Scone with jam, or medium muffin or 4 Jaffa cakes	35
Medium piece of fruit e.g. pear, orange, apple	15
500ml sports drink or squash	30
Lunch	
4 slices bread or medium baked potato	60
150g low fat fruit yoghurt	10
Banana (large) or 50g raisins	35
Snack	
Bagel with honey or jam	50
Medium piece of fruit e.g. pear, orange, apple	15
500ml sports drink or squash	30
Evening meal	
Pasta (250g cooked weight)	80
Broccoli and tomato sauce	20
410g tin of fruit salad	50
150g low fat custard or ice cream	20
500ml squash or diluted juice	30
Snack	
50g chocolate or cereal bar	30
Total carbohydrate	630 grams

NOTE: This selection is not designed to be a complete and balanced diet. It is meant simply to demonstrate the quantities of food providing sufficient carbohydrate. Only foods containing carbohydrate are listed. Carbohydrate values are rounded to the nearest 5 grams.

Table 1 (iii). Example of carbohydrate loading diet

A 90kg athlete would need to eat foods providing 720-900g of carbohydrate per day. For example:

Breakfast	
90g cereal with 300ml semi-skimmed milk	90
4 slices bread or 4 crumpets, with 4 teaspoons of jam	90
250ml orange juice	25
Snack	
Scone with jam, or medium muffin or 4 Jaffa cakes	35
Banana (large) or 50g raisins	35
500ml sports drink or squash	30
Lunch	
4 slices bread or medium baked potato	60
135g tin of baked beans	20
150g low fat fruit yoghurt	10
Medium piece of fruit e.g. pear, orange, apple	15
500ml squash or diluted juice	30
Snack	
Bagel with honey or jam	50
Banana (large) or 50g raisins	35
500ml sports drink or squash	30
Evening meal	
Pasta or rice (300g cooked weight)	100
Broccoli and tomato sauce	25
410g tin of fruit salad	50
150g low fat custard or ice cream	20
500ml squash or diluted juice	30
Snack	
50g chocolate or cereal bar	30
Total carbohydrate	810 grams

NOTE: This selection is not designed to be a complete and balanced diet. It is meant simply to demonstrate the quantities of food providing sufficient carbohydrate. Only foods containing carbohydrate are listed. Carbohydrate values are rounded to the nearest 5 grams.

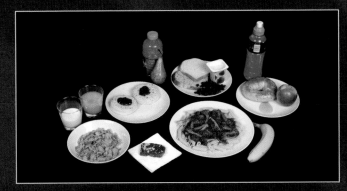

Table 1(i).
A 50kg athlete would need to eat foods providing 400-500g of carbohydrate per day.

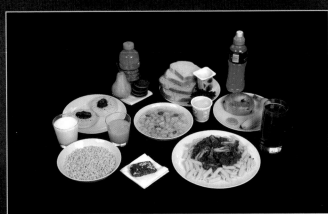

Table 1(ii).
A 70kg athlete would need to eat foods providing 560-700g of carbohydrate per day.

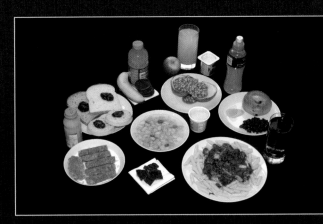

Table 1(iii).
A 90kg athlete would need to eat foods providing 720-900g of carbohydrate per day.

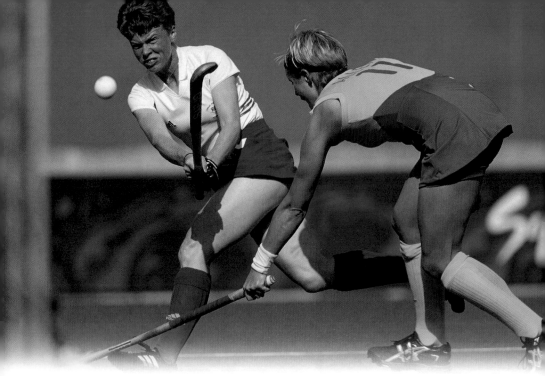

Although carbohydrate loading is mainly thought to be useful for endurance events, such as marathons, triathlons, prolonged cycling and cross-country skiing, it may also enhance performance during intermittent high intensity exercise such as team sports. However, the benefits of carbohydrate loading may be both sport and position specific so it's important to try it out during training to see whether it suits your needs and requirements. What is sure though, is that low carbohydrate stores will impair performance.

Carbohydrate loading has also been shown to increase exercise performance in the heat - so this is something to experiment with in training if the competition takes place in a warmer climate. Furthermore, it's important to add that both male and female athletes will benefit from carbohydrate loading, providing both energy and carbohydrate intakes are also adequate.

Sometimes it is difficult to fully carbohydrate load when competitive events are more than once a week. Nonetheless, it's still important to try to fuel up as much as practically possible and perhaps focus on preparation for the most important competitions - such as the finals.

During carbohydrate loading your carbohydrate requirements will be high and so you will probably need to eat frequent snacks and meals to achieve this. Therefore, you need to look after your teeth by brushing twice a day with a fluoride toothpaste and visiting the dentist regularly.

Pre-Competition Meal

Eating a carbohydrate-rich meal 3-4 hours before exercise can increase glycogen stores, and so is generally thought to enhance exercise performance. The effect may be due to an increase in muscle glycogen stores or liver glycogen stores, but either way it helps maintain blood glucose levels and so improves performance during subsequent exercise. Therefore, pre-competition meals can help stock inadequate muscle glycogen stores and restore liver glycogen stores, which get depleted during the night. Restoring liver glycogen is particularly important for morning competitions.

The focus of the pre-competition meal should be on carbohydrate-rich foods, particularly when stores are inadequate and the event is of sufficient duration and intensity that it is likely to challenge carbohydrate stores. For shorter events, that do not cause fatigue or deplete carbohydrate stores the pre-competition meal does not need to be predominantly carbohydrate. For intense competitions that last longer than an hour, then it is recommended that athletes consume 1-4g carbohydrate per kg body weight during the six hour period before competing.

Table 2 (overleaf) gives seven different examples of pre-competition foods that provide 1-4g carbohydrate per kg body weight for three individuals with different body weights. Very similar foods have been used between the individuals to illustrate what happens to foods and quantities in different circumstances.

You can also design your own pre-competition meals with your favourite foods by using the food charts in fuelling fitness extras. Again it's important to experiment with different foods and amounts during training to find which pre-exercise foods suit you in terms of providing: extra energy; reducing hunger; settling the stomach; and of course being both convenient and practical.

Table 2. Examples of pre-competition meals

(i) A 50kg athlete would need to eat 50-200g carbohydrate. Below are seven different meals each providing about 100g of carbohydrate:

1. 60g cereal with 200ml milk, and large banana or 50g raisins
2. 3 thick slices of bread with honey or jam and 250ml fruit juice
3. Bagel, large banana and 500ml sports drink
4. Baked potato with 135g tin of baked beans and 200ml orange juice
5. 200g pasta with broccoli and tomato sauce and a large apple
6. 100g cous cous with 1/3 can of sweetcorn (100g) and 150ml fruit juice
7. 180g rice with 150g chick peas and medium banana

(ii) A 70kg athlete would need to eat 70-280g carbohydrate. Below are seven different meals each providing about 140g of carbohydrate:

1. 100g cereal with 300ml milk, and large banana or 50g raisins
2. 4 thick slices of bread with honey or jam and 400ml fruit juice
3. 2 Bagels, large banana and 500ml sports drink
4. Baked potato with 270g tin of baked beans and 400ml orange juice
5. 250g pasta with broccoli and tomato sauce and two large apples
6. 125g cous cous with 2/3 can of sweetcorn (200g) and 175ml fruit juice
7. 270g rice with 200g chick peas and large banana

(iii) A 90kg athlete would need to eat 90-360g carbohydrate. Below are seven different meals each providing about 180g of carbohydrate:

1. 150g cereal with 300ml milk, and large banana or 50g raisins
2. 6 thick slices of bread with honey or jam and 400ml fruit juice
3. 2 Bagels, 2 medium bananas and 750ml sports drink
4. 2 Baked potatoes with 270g tin of baked beans and 200ml orange juice
5. 300g pasta with broccoli and tomato sauce plus large banana and apple
6. 150g cous cous with can of sweetcorn (300g) and 200ml fruit juice
7. 360g rice with 250g chick peas and large banana

NOTE: Only foods containing carbohydrate are listed. Carbohydrate values are rounded to the nearest 5 grams.

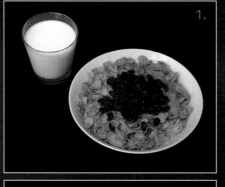

1.

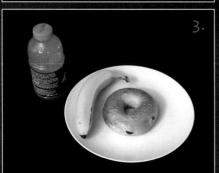

2.

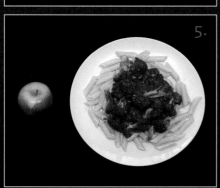

3.

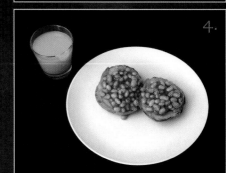

4.

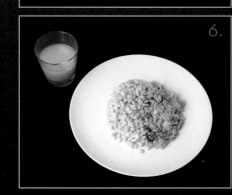

5.

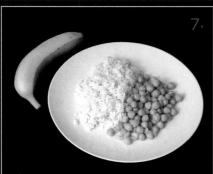

6.

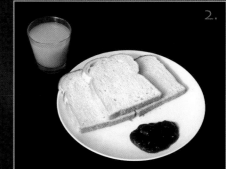

7.

Table 2.
(i) A 50kg athlete would need to eat 50-200g carbohydrate. Shown are seven different meals each providing about 100g of carbohydrate.

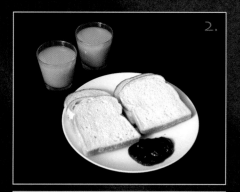

1.

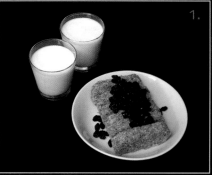

2.

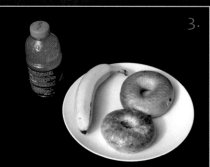

3.

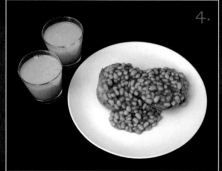

4.

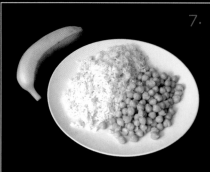

5.

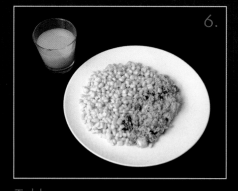

6.

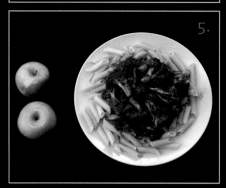

7.

Table 2.

(ii) A 70kg athlete would need to eat 70-280g carbohydrate. Shown are seven different meals each providing about 140g of carbohydrate.

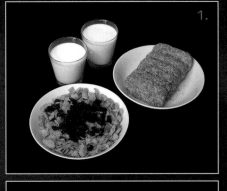

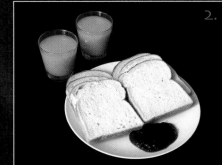

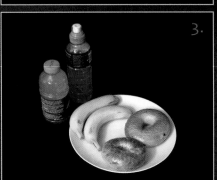

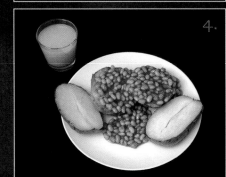

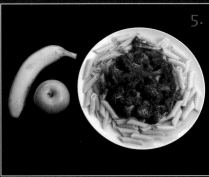

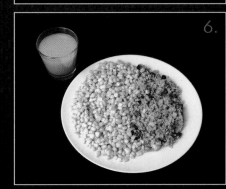

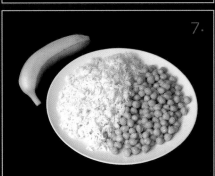

Table 2.

(iii) A 90kg athlete would need to eat 90-360g carbohydrate. Shown are seven different meals each providing about 180g of carbohydrate.

Choosing low GI carbohydrates for the pre-competition meal sometimes helps sustain the delivery of carbohydrate during exercise. However, this does not necessarily improve performance, particularly when additional carbohydrate is consumed during the event. It is not essential that carbohydrate is eaten in the hour or two before competition, providing a carbohydrate loading diet has been followed in the 2-3 days before competition and the event is not late in the day.

Furthermore, when the event is early in the morning, there is not always four hours prior to competing to be able to have a pre-competition meal - and sacrificing sleep to do so is not always the best option! Here, an alternative option would be to have a lighter meal or snack and continue to consume carbohydrate during the event to balance missed fuelling opportunities. This approach may also be useful for individuals who suffer abdominal discomfort when they consume large quantities of food. It is also advisable to choose foods for pre-competition meals that are low fat, low fibre and low to moderate protein, as they are less likely to cause stomach upsets. Liquid meal supplements or carbohydrate-containing drinks and bars are also

particularly useful for athletes who get a bad attack of the nerves prior to competing.

Carbohydrates Immediately Before and During Exercise

Although it is a good idea to allow 2-4 hours after a large meal before exercising, a high carbohydrate snack 30-60 minutes before exercise can be beneficial for some individuals, providing enough carbohydrate is eaten without unnecessary abdominal discomfort.

Generally, ingestion of carbohydrate in the hour prior to exercise does not impair exercise performance, except in susceptible individuals. However, there are no clear signals of susceptibility to rebound hypoglycaemia (low blood glucose levels) during exercise and so this should be assessed by individual experience during training.

If pre-exercise carbohydrate is the only means of increasing carbohydrate availability during exercise, then it is important that a substantial amount of carbohydrate - ideally more than 70g - is eaten. The main problem with pre-competition meals is when too little carbohydrate -

less than 50g - is eaten followed by none during the event. This small amount of carbohydrate sets the body up to rely on carbohydrates for fuel, but doesn't supply enough to sustain the exercise.

It is best to opt for a high GI carbohydrate, although if carbohydrate is going to be eaten during prolonged exercise the GI of the pre-exercise snack is not so important. And, indeed, some athletes may prefer and be more at home with low GI carbohydrates. However, it is probably advisable to avoid the more bulky (fibre-rich) carbohydrates, as these can cause abdominal discomfort. (See section on fuelling training and recovery for further information on GI)

If carbohydrates are eaten immediately before exercise or during rest periods in prolonged exercise - lasting more than 40 minutes - it is sometimes beneficial to continue to ingest 30-60g carbohydrate per hour throughout exercise to help maintain the flow of glucose.

During exercise that lasts for longer than an hour and which brings about fatigue, it is advisable to consume 30-60g per hour of rapidly absorbed carbohydrate, because it generally improves performance. This intake is best achieved by taking feedings every 10-30min, depending on what's allowed by the event, and should be continued throughout the event so that it provides a steady flow of glucose into the blood-stream.

Carbohydrate ingestion in the day and hours before exercise and during exercise has interactive effects. It's vital that you plan and practise fuelling strategies for competition during training to find out what suits you, as well as what is allowed within the rules of your sport. During important competitions is not the time to try out new foods or fuelling strategies! Further information can be found in the section on fuelling training and recovery - plus see Table 7 in that section for some ideas of pre-exercise snacks that provide at least 50g of carbohydrate.

Increased Fat Availability

Another potential strategy to enhance endurance exercise performance is to increase fat availability. In doing so it is hoped that carbohydrate utilization will be reduced and so delay the onset of carbohydrate depletion and fatigue. Increasing fat availability prior to exercise - in hours as well as acutely before exercise - does help reduce carbohydrate utilization during subsequent exercise, but this does not seem to enhance exercise performance. Therefore, a period of 'fat adaptation' - around 5 days - does not seem to provide any additional benefit.

However, it's still early days research wise. So, if fat adaptation can be shown to be an effective strategy for enhancing performance in some athletes, then most will find that a brief exposure is more practical, and better tolerated, than a prolonged period of increased dietary fat intake. Besides, following a high fat diet for too long a period displaces carbohydrate intake and so will ultimately affect exercise performance. Therefore, increased fat availability is best thought of as a pre-competition tactic rather than a long-term training strategy. However, it should be experimented with during training to discover whether it suits you and improves performance - the ultimate outcome.

Hydrating Prior to Competition

Since it is likely that some degree of dehydration will occur during competition, it is vital that athletes are well hydrated prior to competing. Therefore, pre-competition preparation should also consider hydration levels to ensure fluid and salt losses from previous training sessions or competition, or from 'making-weight' attempts for weight category sports, have been optimally replaced.

Hydration strategies are an important aspect of pre-competition planning and are discussed in more detail in the section on liquids. Athletes should drink sufficient fluid the day before competition to ensure that they are well hydrated. Some athletes attempt to over-hydrate prior to competing to help avoid the inevitable detrimental fluid losses that are likely to occur during the event or because of the environmental conditions for the event. However, this should previously be tested out during hard training sessions that mimic the competitive situation.

Even if you aren't trying to over-hydrate there are still good reasons to drink in the hours before exercise. Prior to competition it is recommended to drink around 400-600ml of fluid with or without carbohydrate, depending on individual circumstances, in the 60-90 minute period before competing. This will not only help ensure adequate hydration levels, but also allows enough time to pee out any excess fluids prior to competing. It is also beneficial to drink 300-500ml of fluid in the 10-15 minutes prior to strenuous events that last longer than an hour.

Again, it's fundamental that you plan and practise hydrating strategies that you intend to adopt before, during and after competition, during training sessions to find out what suits you, as well as what is allowed within the rules of your sport. As always it is not advisable to try out new drinks or hydration strategies during important competitions!

Recovery

Remember, as in training, to sustain competition and compete again - be it in a few hours, the next day or in a week's time - you must recover sufficiently by resting, restocking glycogen stores and replacing fluid and salt losses.

Turn to the sections on fuelling training and recovery and liquid assets for further information on recovery strategies.

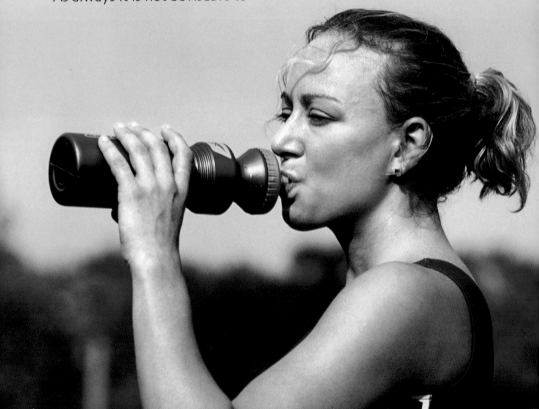

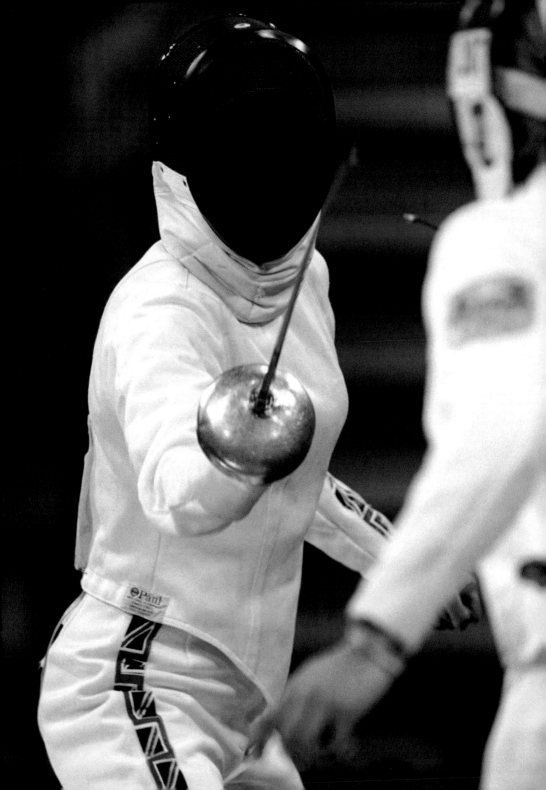

8

Supplementary Thoughts

≈ **Dietary supplement use in sport is widespread**

≈ **The majority of supplements are ineffective**

≈ **Supplementing the diet does not make a bad diet better**

≈ **Excessive intake of some supplements can do more harm than good**

≈ **Indiscriminate use of supplements is unwise due to potential health, contamination and doping risks**

Supplements come in many forms and guises and their use in sport is widespread. If you eat a varied, well-balanced diet that meets the energy demands of your training do you really need to supplement your diet? Banned or not, are supplements safe, cost effective and do they actually work?

The use of supplements in sport is widespread. A supplement simply does just that - it supplements the diet. The role of diet in supporting athletic training becomes even more important when training levels - intensity, duration and frequency - are high. Previous sections of this book have looked at the way diet can be optimized to support training levels to lead to enhanced exercise and competitive performance. Informed dietary choices can ensure fuel needs are met to promote:

- Adaptations to training

- Recovery so that training can be continued and intensified

- Good health to help prevent illness and injury

A varied, well-balanced diet that meets the energy demands of training should provide adequate amounts of all the essential nutrients. However, sometimes this is not possible. And indeed, in some situations, obtaining sufficient amounts from the diet is often not so straightforward. Consequently, many athletes take dietary supplements in the hope that it will compensate for poor food choices and make up for vital nutrients that they feel are lacking in their diet.

Supplement Usage

Surveys show that nearly half of all athletes use supplements - of course their popularity varies widely between different sports and between athletes of differing ages, performance levels, and cultural backgrounds. In some sports, particularly strength and power sports, supplement usage is so common it is perceived as normal. But, that does not mean it should be the norm! And, besides, many athletes would benefit from improving their diet rather than resorting to taking an inappropriate supplement. Simply taking a supplement does not necessarily make up for a bad diet!

Not only is supplement usage common, but all too often the recommended doses are exceeded. Sometimes it is simply an attempt to outdo what their opponent is taking. However, more does not necessarily mean better, and in the case of some supplements - such as the fat-soluble vitamins (A, D, E and K) and iron - more can be toxic, and so would actually be doing more harm than good.

The frequently quoted reasons for supplement use include:

- Compensation for an inadequate diet

- To meet unusual demands of hard training or competition

- To produce specific benefits to exercise performance

- To keep up with team-mates or opponents

- Recommended by coach, parent or other influential individuals

It's important to note that the decision to use supplements is not always a rational one. Even when athletes are informed that the diet is sufficient or that nutrient status of their body's stores is normal (for example iron stores) they still continue to take supplements as perhaps a form of insurance - 'just in case'.

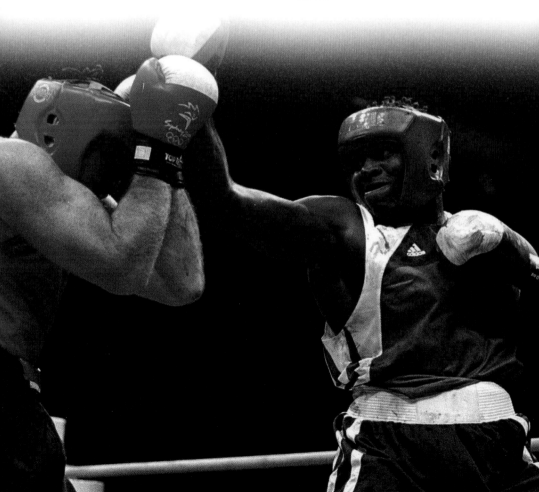

Common Supplements

The list of supplements and ergogenic aids used within the exercise environment is exhaustive. Supplements also come in many forms and guises. Table 1 gives a list of the types of commonly used sports nutrition supplements.

Special sports foods, including energy bars and sports drinks have a genuine role to play in supplementing the training diet. Some common protein supplements and liquid meal replacements may also be useful in certain situations.

In some instances, where there is an established deficiency of an essential nutrient, supplementing the diet with food or dietary supplements to correct the deficiency can be beneficial, but, again exceeding the nutrient requirements is not necessarily

Table 1. Common sports nutrition supplements

Sports drinks
Carbohydrate bars and gels
Protein powders, drinks and bars
Liquid meal supplements
Vitamin and mineral supplements
Ergogenic aids

a good thing. Nutrient supplements and drinks, in particular carbohydrate and protein, as well as vitamin, mineral and antioxidant supplements are covered specifically in separate sections of this book.

Ergogenic aids are substances that aim to enhance performance through effects on energy, alertness, or body composition. Athletes are forever searching for that magic bullet that will improve performance and give them a competitive edge, but is not against the rules! Even if a supplement does all that, it could still be harmful in the short or long term.

In this section we will focus on the commonly used legal supplements where there is enough scientific

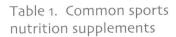

evidence to suggest that they may have potential benefits in certain situations.

Energy

Several nutritional ergogenic aids are effective at influencing energy supply. The most obvious example is carbohydrate supplements - whether in the form of powders, gels or sports drinks. Carbohydrates during prolonged exercise provide extra energy fuel to help prevent fatigue. Sports drinks deliver water and fuel to the body fast - so help to avoid dehydration and fatigue.

Several other ergogenic aids have been shown to be potentially beneficial for certain athletes. In particular, creatine and bicarbonate supplements have been demonstrated to be useful during high intensity work. However, the long term effects are still unclear, so unless you're competing at the top level, they are probably not worth the risk or indeed the financial cost!

Creatine

In the first few seconds or so of sprint exercise, creatine phosphate is used as a fuel. (See section on energy) Creatine supplementation can increase muscle creatine phosphate levels and therefore may be useful to help athletes recover quickly between repeated bouts of high intensity exercise. Creatine supplementation may also result in an increase in muscle mass, which is not necessarily useful for all athletes.

Typically a non-vegetarian diet provides about 1g of creatine a day - vegetarians will get virtually no creatine from their diet. However, not many strength and power athletes, where creatine is perhaps more important, are vegetarian! So it's questionable whether it is the high meat content or the creatine that is the important component of the diet.

Creatine supplementation has generally been shown to be effective at improving performance. However, the supplement dosage is often high - usually around 20g per day for 4-5 days (a loading dose) followed by 1-2g per day (a maintenance dose) - and so it is far more than you could realistically get from your diet. So it is not possible to say simply increase your intake of meat and fish to match these dosage levels! However, exceeding this maximum effective dosage is not helpful and may actually be harmful.

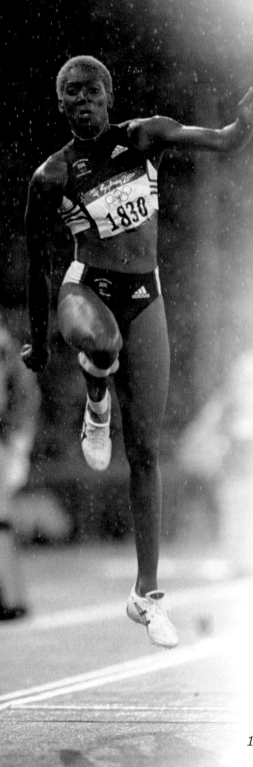

Bicarbonate

During high intensity exercise the muscles produce lactic acid, which can cause pain and interfere with exercise performance. For the same reason that many people use antacids to neutralize excess stomach acidity, alkaline salts, such as sodium bicarbonate (baking soda), can help to neutralize the acidity of lactic acid in the muscles and thereby delay the onset of fatigue.

Taking some bicarbonate - around 0.3g per kg body weight, so that's about 24g for an 80kg athlete - over a period of 2-3 hours before exercise can improve performance in events lasting a few minutes. However, the usefulness of bicarbonate is restricted to short-term high-intensity exercise with benefits being unlikely in events that last longer than 10 minutes.

Some susceptible individuals experience gastrointestinal side-effects such as vomiting and diarrhoea with high doses of bicarbonate. For most the effects are not severe, and certainly not serious, and also disappear as tolerance develops. Other acid-neutralizing substances, such as sodium citrate, may be equally effective and generally produce fewer side-effects.

Stimulants

The list of substances prohibited in competitive sport includes stimulants. However, caffeine is unique in that it is a central nervous system (CNS) stimulant but is commonly consumed in a wide range of food and drinks. Caffeine also has a direct effect on muscles and adipose tissue (fat). In particular it is believed to mobilize fatty acids from adipose tissue stores, increasing the availability of fat as a fuel during exercise, which in-turn helps spare the limited glycogen (carbohydrate) stores and extend exercise time.

Caffeine contained in commonly available beverages can enhance power output during the later stages of prolonged endurance exercise and may also be helpful in short-term high-intensity exercise. This benefit can be obtained with relatively small doses of caffeine - about 1.5mg/kg body weight so that's about 100mg for a 70kg athlete - from commonly consumed drinks such as coffee and cola beverages.

Recently, attention has focused on caffeine's effect on the CNS. Several studies have found that caffeine is performance enhancing during exercise of varying duration and intensities - so that's most sports - at low doses of less than 5mg/kg body weight and perhaps as low as 3mg/kg body weight. This suggests that its main effect is on the CNS. This implies that caffeine at low doses can enhance exercise performance during both training and competition. Furthermore, during training, the ability to be able to train harder could also lead to better training adaptations.

Although caffeine is a drug, and so will produce different effects on different people, these low doses are unlikely to cause any health problems. The sensitivity to caffeine varies enormously between individuals, but does not seem to be related to the habitual amount of caffeine consumed. Caffeine can produce limiting side-effects in some individuals such as insomnia, headaches and abdominal discomfort, as well as muscle tremors and impaired coordination at high doses. Therefore, as always, it is important to experiment with caffeine during training, before contemplating using it during competition. Caffeine is also a mild diuretic so it is important to make sure you stay well hydrated, particularly if consuming caffeine in a tablet form, or during prolonged endurance exercise, or when exercising in a hot and humid environment.

Prior to January 2004, a caffeine level in the urine above 12mg/l was not permitted during competition and would result in a positive drug test. In general, this level was achieved by taking about 500mg caffeine - that's about 6 cups of strong coffee - in a short time. Although caffeine is indeed a drug (that is weakly addictive) it is both socially acceptable and unrealistic to try to control it. Therefore, due to the wide-availability of caffeine in drinks and foods, it is difficult, but not impossible to have a caffeine intake level that exceeds the permissible limit just from a normal diet. See Table 2 for the caffeine content of some common drinks. Primarily as a result of this, the World Anti-Doping Agency (WADA) decided to remove caffeine from the list of banned substances with effect from January 2004.

Table 2.
Caffeine content
of common drinks

Standard drink	Caffeine content (mg)
Instant coffee	50-70
Filter coffee	60-120
Tea	15-50
Hot chocolate	8-15
Cola	20-50

Body Composition

A variety of supplements claim to enhance performance by affecting body composition - either by increasing muscle mass and/or reducing body fat. Supplements within this broad category include protein and amino acid supplements, carnitine, chromium, hydroxymethylbutyrate (HMB), as well as boron, chrysin, colostrum, creatine, ornithine, alphaketoglutarate, tribulus terrestris, vanadium and zinc. However, most have been shown to be ineffective. Protein and amino acids supplements are covered specifically in the section on protein.

Furthermore, there is no evidence that taking prohormones such as androstenedione ('andro') and norandrostenedione results in a significant increase in blood testosterone nor are they effective at increasing muscle size or strength. In addition, these supplements may pose serious health risks, and also result in positive drug test in the sports in which their usage is banned.

Immune Function

Both heavy exercise and nutrition produce separate influences on immune function. Although modest exercise is good for the immune system, very strenuous and prolonged training is associated with a depressed immune function. An inadequate diet or inappropriate food choices on top of hard training will further depress immune function.

Dietary deficiencies of energy, carbohydrate, protein and certain micronutrients, in particular iron, zinc and vitamins A, E, B6 and B12, will impair immune function. Although athletes need to avoid nutrient deficiencies by adapting their diet, it is also important not to exceed requirements of both dietary fat, in particular omega-3 (η-3) fatty acids, and some micronutrients, especially iron, zinc and vitamin E, as this can also have a detrimental effect on immune function.

Although, the effect of hard training on immune function is generally fairly small, any injury or illness that interrupts training or prevents an athlete competing is pretty disastrous to the individual concerned. Consequently, several supplements such as high doses of antioxidant vitamins, glutamine, zinc, probiotics and *Echinacea* are promoted as being 'immune-boosting', but there is no strong evidence that any of these are effective. Currently, the best evidence supports the need for a carbohydrate-rich diet, which lowers stress hormone levels, along with adequate rest periods. In addition, it appears to be beneficial to consume about 30-60g of carbohydrate per hour during prolonged exercise since this will help reduce some of the negative effects of prolonged exercise.

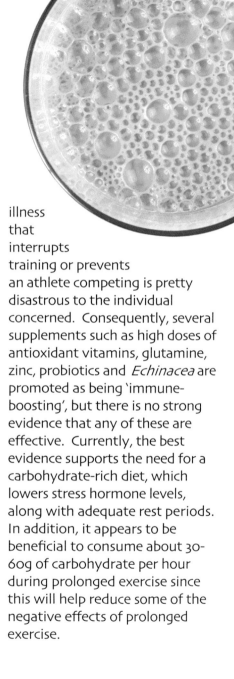

Joint Health

Many supplements are promoted as being good for joint health, by reducing the wear and tear caused by overuse such as strenuous training. The main supplements promoted for joint health include: antioxidants; fatty acids; vitamins B3, B5 and D; calcium; boron; proteolytic enzymes; glucosamine, chondroitin, methylsulphonylmethane (MSM); S-Adenosyl methionine (SaME); type 2 collagen; hyaluronic acid; and soy isoflavones. However, most have been shown to be ineffective.

Healthy bones need an adequate supply of calcium and vitamin D, but these are normally supplied from a healthy balanced diet and so supplementation is generally not necessary.

There is also some evidence that regular (once or twice a day) long-term (about 2-6 months) treatment with glucosamine and chondroitin sulphate can provide subjective relief in individuals with osteoarthritis. However, there is currently no evidence that this would also be beneficial to athletes with joint pain.

Contamination Issues

As a result of poor manufacturing practice, some products have been shown to contain impurities such as lead, broken glass and animal faeces. Some products have been found not to contain the expensive ingredients listed on the label, but only inexpensive materials. And some products contain banned doping agents such as steroid hormones, for example nandrolone and testosterone, that are not supposed to be there.

One survey by the IOC laboratory in Cologne found that at least 1 in 7, and possibly as high as 1 in 4, of the products they analysed contained steroid hormones and their precursors - these would cause an athlete to fail a drug test. Substantial numbers of positive tests were obtained from dietary supplements bought in the UK (19%), The Netherlands (26%) and the USA (19%).

However, due to the inadequate regulation of dietary supplements, there is no way for consumers to know what many supplements actually contain or how pure the product and its ingredients are. In addition, the principle of strict liability means that the onus is on the athlete to be sure - you are responsible for everything you eat and drink. Therefore, athletes who are liable for drug testing under national or international programmes should be extremely cautious about using supplements and always check with a sports doctor before taking any supplements.

Cost and Benefits of Supplements

The indiscriminate use of dietary supplements is unwise due to the very real health and contamination risks. Before deciding to use a dietary supplement it may be useful to think through a cost and benefits process, balancing the potential benefits against the detrimental costs. What are the costs to you in terms of financial, adverse effects on health and sports performance, and the likelihood of contamination with banned substances? Are there any benefits such as improved sports performance, 'insurance policy' against an inadequate diet, better health and are free samples available?

Of course it's not always possible to complete a thorough analysis on every supplement as it is likely that there will be some unknown factors - especially if no scientific research has been carried out on the supplement or its proposed active ingredients.

It is essential to find positive reasons for using a supplement that can be backed-up by a substantial amount of scientific evidence. The evidence for a true benefit must be very strong to outweigh all the potential risks. And not forgetting the powerful placebo effect - just because you believe taking it is going to make you feel good, doesn't mean it actually does!

Finally, avoid dietary 'assessments' that are designed to find faults in your diet that can only be corrected by taking supplements. Supplements are a more efficient way of making a profit than encouraging you to eat a healthy balanced diet. As to whether they will improve sports performance, is another matter!

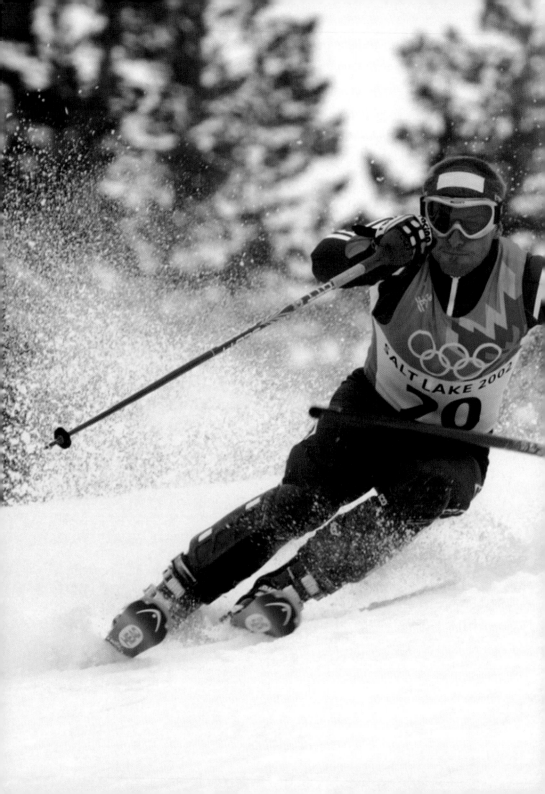

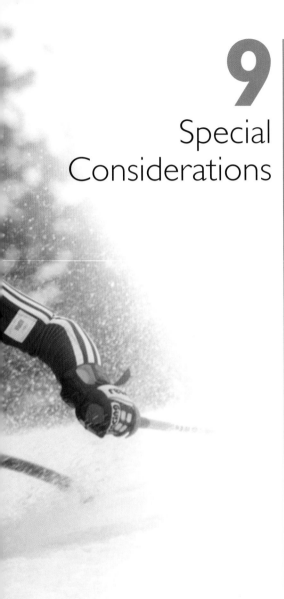

9

Special Considerations

(i)
Endurance Sports
by Penny Hunking

Endurance events seriously challenge athletes' fuel and fluid stores and the longer and more intense the event the more stores deplete. Optimal fuelling before endurance events is crucial. Athletes who pay attention to what they eat and drink before the start are likely to have the edge over those who do not. Even with good nutrition planning athletes can become fatigued during the event and so it is important to consider nutrition strategies that can help reduce and/or delay fatigue.

Nutrition Issues and Solutions

Carbohydrate
A key goal of nutritional strategies prior to exercise is to maximize glycogen stores. Athletes should aim to achieve carbohydrate intakes to meet the fuel requirements of their training programmes, and also adequately replace their carbohydrate stores during recovery between training sessions and competition. Increased dietary carbohydrate in the 2-3 days before exercise is generally associated with enhanced performance. Endurance athletes must eat a diet high in carbohydrate. Carbohydrate is contained in many foods and drinks and carbohydrate supplements such as gels and liquid meals may be useful. Typically a fuel intake of around 20-60g/h is suitable for very long endurance events.

Fluid
Athletes need to be fully hydrated prior to starting exercise and water can be drunk in addition to food or sports drinks to contribute to fluid needs. Athletes should drink regularly throughout exercise lasting more than an hour to limit fluid losses. Isotonic sports drinks can help fluid replacement, whilst also delivering some carbohydrate. Sugary drinks and fruit juices lack sodium and their carbohydrate content may be a little high when fast rehydration is required.

Protein

Protein can be used as an energy source and the amount of protein needed is dependent upon total energy intake and so it is important to eat enough food and calories. Athletes with restricted energy intake may need to take care to consume adequate protein.

Timing of meals and snacks

Regular meals and snacks are necessary in order to pack in the volume of food that is needed to fuel training and competition. For fast refuelling, meals and snacks high in carbohydrate should be eaten as soon as exercise finishes.

Quantity and type of foods eaten

A substantial high carbohydrate meal (as much as 200-300g carbohydrate) should be eaten 3-4 hours before exercise. Carbohydrate intake after exhaustive exercise should average 50g of carbohydrate every two hours of mostly moderate and high Glycaemic Index (GI) foods.

Fibre

It is difficult to eat enough carbohydrate if bulky, fibrous foods are eaten so focus on eating more low fibre and compact foods.

Recovery

It is vital to refuel glycogen stores and replace the fluid and electrolytes lost in sweat. Athletes should start eating and drinking as soon as training and competition has finished if recovery time is limited i.e. less than 8 hours before the next training session.

Experimentation

All dietary strategies should be practised in training to find which suits the athlete best. Athletes should stick to their tried and tested routines and food choices and never try anything new in competition.

Practical Tips and Ideas

Cram in the carbs!

Base meals on bread, rice, pasta, cereals and potatoes

Eat plenty of snacks such as bananas, oranges, dried fruit, jelly beans, honey or jam sandwiches, bagels, sports/muesli/energy bars, chocolate, biscuits e.g. Jaffa cakes, Garibaldi and fig rolls

Drink low fat milk/milkshakes and smoothies

Eat cartons/tins of low fat rice pudding and custard with fruit as a snack or dessert

Carbohydrate gels and liquid meals may be helpful if the athlete is finding it difficult to eat enough food and doesn't want too much food in their stomach

And remember the drinks!

Drink to limit fluid losses during training and competition

Drinks might include: water, isotonic sports drinks, fruit juice, cordial or squash diluted according to manufacturers' instructions, sugary drinks

Key Points

≈ Plan nutrition strategies for competition and start 7 days in advance

≈ Taper exercise in the carbohydrate loading phase

≈ Practise eating and drinking strategies in training to find out what suits

≈ Be aware of the environment and adjust fluid intake to suit the situation

(ii)
Team Sports
by Jane Griffin

Team sports invariably involve repeated bouts of high intensity exercise, both during training and matches, which can seriously deplete carbohydrate stores. Opportunities to take on board fluids during matches are limited by the rules and regulations of the sport. There may be a need to adjust body composition through training and diet to achieve a higher 'power to mass' ratio.

Nutrition Issues and Solutions

Reduced stores of carbohydrate may contribute to fatigue and loss of both physical and mental performance, particularly towards the end of a match or training session. (Many goals or tries are scored in the dying moments of a match.) Players with reduced stores of carbohydrate are at greater risk of injury. All types of training will reduce stores to some extent so players must refuel immediately after every training session when recovery time is limited.

Players should start all training sessions and matches well-hydrated. The warmer and more humid the weather the more players will sweat but training hard on cold days also results in sweat losses. Players must take every opportunity offered during training and matches to drink and rehydrate effectively with the right sort of fluid. Ideally the drink should be isotonic containing carbohydrate and salt, and athletes should use this in preference to water because of its advantages to performance. Some players need to 'bulk-up' while others must reduce body fat. Players who need to increase muscle mass must eat regularly, often fitting in 5-6 meals of varying size into the day, including post-training intake of carbohydrate and protein. Often those who need to 'bulk-up' are the ones least interested in food and they must work hard at their diet. Rest, recovery and patience are the other key factors in encouraging 'bulking-up'. Players who need to lose body fat must be aware of fat in their diet, especially hidden fats.

Practical Tips and Ideas

Take suitable snacks and drinks in the kit bag
Start refuelling as soon after training/competition as possible - ideally in the changing room - if recovery time is limited
Use rest days to eat appropriately and make-up any shortfalls in the diet
Eating late at night (e.g. baked beans on toast) after evening training is better than not eating at all
Don't be traditional! Eat sandwiches for breakfast and cereal as a late-night snack if that suits better
A freezer and microwave are invaluable and considerably cut down on shopping, preparation and cooking time
Use available opportunities to drink appropriate fluids during training and matches
Include protein with carbohydrate after 'bulking-up' training sessions
Be alert to the hidden fat in food
Seek professional advice before taking any supplements

Key Points

≈ Team sports can seriously deplete carbohydrate stores

≈ There may be a need to adjust body composition through training and diet to achieve a higher 'power to mass' ratio

≈ Players must refuel after every training session

≈ Players must take available opportunities offered during training and matches to drink

≈ Carrying fluid and snacks in the kit bag is important

(iii)
Strength, Power and Sprint Sports
by Karen Reid

The main role of nutrition for strength, power and sprint athletes is to support the development of lean body mass, reduce and control body fat levels, and meet the energy demands of the training programme.

Nutrition Issues and Solutions

Carbohydrate

It is a common myth amongst this group of athletes that carbohydrates are 'fattening' and should be restricted or even avoided at certain times of the day.

However, whilst the carbohydrate requirements of strength, power and sprint athletes are not as great as endurance athletes, research has shown that a sufficient intake of carbohydrate is essential for maintaining strength training volume and muscular endurance.

A low carbohydrate diet has also been shown to impair high intensity anaerobic performance. Depending on the phase of training typically between 5-7g carbohydrate per kg body mass per day is an appropriate intake.

It is recommended that carbohydrate with a high Glycaemic Index (GI) is consumed within 1 hour after training for speedy recovery. Between 0.5-1.5g carbohydrate per kg body mass should be taken depending on the intensity and duration of the session.

Beneficial effects of carbohydrate post exercise include:

- Stimulation of insulin secretion after training

- Enhanced muscle glycogen resynthesis

- Improved amino acid uptake

- Promotion of an anabolic hormonal environment post-training

- Plus carbohydrate appears to reduce the breakdown of muscle tissue

Combining protein and carbohydrate post-training

Combining some protein with carbohydrate after training promotes an anabolic hormonal environment and increases net protein synthesis. That is it helps promote the development of muscle.

The amount of protein required is quite modest and a carbohydrate based snack or drink containing between 10 - 20g of protein is sufficient for most athletes followed by a balanced meal 1-2 hours later containing both carbohydrate and protein. (See suggestions below)

The composition of a number of the protein shakes marketed at this group of athletes is not ideal as they typically contain very low amounts of carbohydrate and have protein levels which are in excess of 20g per serving.

Optimizing carbohydrate and protein intake

It is important that strength, power and sprint athletes avoid excessive intakes of protein from protein shakes and supplements. In most cases an adequate protein intake can be achieved from food, and there is no evidence that the quality of protein from supplements is superior to food sources.

Protein intakes in excess of requirements won't help build muscle, and would be better replaced with carbohydrate foods before and after training to ensure good energy reserves.

Practical Tips and Ideas

The following food and drink suggestions are ideal choices for promoting optimum recovery and protein synthesis after training, by providing both carbohydrate and 10-20g of protein:

Low fat flavoured milk or yoghurt drinks e.g. skimmed milk mixed with milkshake flavour, or bananas and honey liquidized with low fat milk

Cereal and low fat milk

200g low fat yoghurt with 75g dried fruit

500ml of sports drink and a sandwich with a protein filling e.g. chicken, ham, egg, low fat cheese or tuna

Key Points

≈ **Most strength and power athletes believe their food focus should be protein**

≈ **Excessive intakes of protein (over 2g per kg per day) are not necessary**

≈ **Essential to start each workout well fuelled and well hydrated**

≈ **Important to optimize recovery by eating a source of protein and carbohydrate immediately before or after the workout**

≈ **Supplement use is discouraged due to doping and contamination issues**

(iv)
Weight Category and Aesthetic Sports
by Gill Horgan

Athletes often want to decrease body weight to compete in a specific weight category, or because they compete in an aesthetic sport, or where they feel that a lower weight may help to increase speed.

Rapid and short term weight loss is often achieved over the few days leading up to an event using techniques such as dehydration and food restriction. Athletes who use this weight loss/gain or 'weight-cycling' find their weight is never stable. They also find that weight often increases over time and is harder to lose each time. For some competitors this can lead to many bizarre eating habits or even eating disorders.

Nutrition Issues and Solutions

If weight loss is necessary and appropriate, it is good practice to begin the process well in advance of the competitive season.

Long term management ideals:

- Limit the amount of weight that must be lost at the last minute

- Avoid resorting to rapid weight loss techniques (dehydration through excess sweating or voluntarily restricting fluid intake, starvation or self imposed laxative or diuretic abuse and vomiting)

- Avoid loss of lean body mass, body water and muscle glycogen (which will affect performance)

- Avoid maintaining too low a body weight or body fat levels which are inappropriately low (which increases the risk of developing eating disorders)

- Avoid weight-cycling, which may lead to a decrease in resting metabolic rate; altered body composition (increased ratio of fat to lean tissue); altered fat deposition (greater abdominal fat); altered hormone profiles and possible nutrient deficiencies

Genetics play a role in determining body fat levels. Athletes should seek professional advice from a sports nutrition expert, such as a sports dietitian or registered sport and exercise nutritionist, to identify the ideal body fat/weight goal which is consistent with long term health and good performance. It is important to have an eating plan which meets these goals.

The body lays down 0.5kg of fat for every additional 3,500 calories that are eaten above the body's energy requirements during a week. So to lose 0.5kg of weight a week, cut 500 calories from the daily diet.

Practical Tips and Ideas

Try to eat balanced meals regularly including all the food groups, but avoiding high fat foods

Try to eat/drink some carbohydrate after training

Drink to maintain good hydration. For every 0.5kg (1lb) lost during training you need to drink 500ml to replace fluid levels and another 250ml for extra sweating - so drink 1.5 x weight loss to cover each session

It can take up to 24 hours or longer to fully hydrate after a period of dehydration

Drink after weigh-in

Weigh-in shortly before event

Drink an isotonic sports drink which will help replace fluid and carbohydrate stores

Weigh-in the morning before evening event

Isotonic drink, light, high carbohydrate meal and snacks

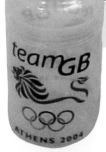

Key Points

≈ **Choose a body weight/body fat level which is achievable and healthy**

≈ **Do not crash diet, dehydrate or follow bizarre eating patterns**

≈ **If you need to lose weight have a plan which allows gradual reduction in weight (fat) levels (not more than 0.5-1.0kg (1-2lbs) per week) or 2-5mm of fat if using skinfold measurements**

≈ **This can normally be achieved by reducing energy intake by 500 kcals per day. It is important to ensure adequate energy and nutrient intake for training**

≈ **Athletes should not reduce energy intake too low. Supervision by a sports nutrition expert such as a sports dietitian or registered sport and exercise nutritionist is recommended**

≈ **Do not train at more than 2-3kg (4.4-6.6lbs) away from competition weight**

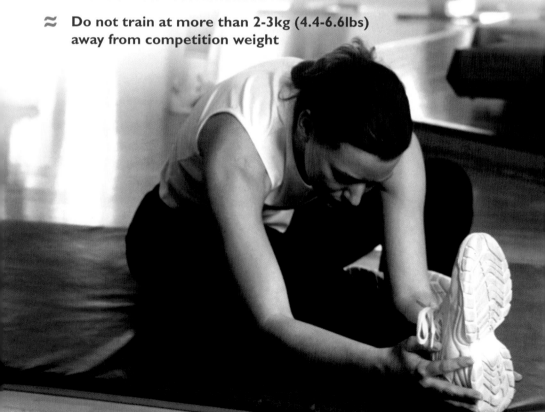

(v)
Winter Sports
by Marianne Hayward
and Jan Masson

The many different winter sports events, e.g. biathlon, skiing (alpine, cross-country, downhill, mogul, slalom, super-G), ski-jumping, curling, luge, ice-skating, bobsleigh, skeleton, speed skating, ice hockey and snowboarding vary in intensity and energy demands. Consequently the nutritional needs of the individual athlete will be equally diverse. Whatever the competitive event optimum fuel reserves and hydration are important.

Winter athletes often have to travel and train abroad for long periods - affecting their eating and drinking habits. Preparation and planning in advance, together with sensible menu choices of foods, aids optimal nutritional strategies for training and competition.

Additional nutritional issues for Winter sport athletes include the special needs arising from the environment in which they are often undertaken, including extreme cold and high altitude. This can result in a greater physical stress compared to similar exercise at sea level, which can limit their ability to train or compete.

Nutrition Issues and Solutions

Energy

Training requirements of male cross-country skiers can be in the region of 6000-8000 calories per day. Keeping-up with energy and carbohydrate requirements can be quite challenging. Downhill skiers, speed skaters and ice dancers may be striving for lower body fat levels for improving power to weight ratios, or for aesthetic appearances. Failure to meet energy demands can lead to weight loss, poor recovery and under-performance. Curlers require sufficient energy to sustain long competitions of up to 2.5-3 hours and may have two games a day.

135

Training and competing at altitude depresses appetite. Nutrition strategies must include small meals and regular snacks to compensate.

Carbohydrate

Training and competing at altitude, results in an increased dependence on glucose, as a fuel, both at rest and during exercise. How much will depend on the intensity of the sport. Cross country skiers will require up to 10g per kg body weight, whereas curlers will require closer to 6-7g per kg body weight.

Refuelling after training or an event should be a priority, but often other things get in the way e.g. looking after equipment, being first on the lift, travelling to and from the mountain. It is essential therefore to have compact snacks such as dried fruit, cereal bars, low fat milkshakes, jelly sweets and low fat biscuits that do not deteriorate in the cold, and can easily be carried in pockets, food bags or rucksacks.

Fluid

Exposure to cold reduces the sensation of thirst and there is a reduced voluntary intake of fluids. It is therefore vitally important to ensure practical strategies are in place to promote more frequent consumption of appropriate volumes and types of drinks. Weighing before and after practice sessions may be an effective way of assessing sweat losses. Isotonic sports drinks are widely available and a good choice. Dehydration can reduce mental awareness, which is important to avoid, especially in a strategic sport such as curling. However, in temperatures of -15°C and below, in driving sleet or with wind gusts that add a substantial wind chill factor, freezing cold drinks rapidly lose their appeal.

Practical Tips and Ideas

Make flasks of hot liquids e.g. hot blackcurrant or lemon, or pasta/rice/potato based soups

Hot drinks have a 'feel good' factor and can help the body save heat

Isotonic sports drinks can be useful for facilitating refuelling as well as hydration

Fluid should be taken on board throughout competition and training

Key Points

≈ Training and competing in the cold/altitude increases energy, in particular carbohydrate, requirements

≈ Appetite will be suppressed in the cold/altitude therefore energy dense carbohydrate snacks should be eaten throughout training and competition

≈ Carbohydrate foods such as dried fruit, milkshakes, jelly sweets and cereal bars are useful. Warm soups based on rice, potatoes and pasta are easily digestible and may provide a 'feel good' factor

≈ Pay attention to fluid intake, particularly at higher altitudes

≈ Winter sports are associated with a greater risk of injury and accidents, so it is important to avoid fatigue by maintaining adequate fuel and fluid status

≈ Foods that are rich in antioxidants, such as a variety of fruit and vegetables, may also be useful to help combat the extra physical stress experienced at altitude

(vi)
Disability Sport
by Jeanette Crosland

There are a range of disability classifications in sport. The major principles of sports nutrition can be applied to all athletes whether able bodied or disabled. It is essential that all athletes eat a diet which provides the right amount of carbohydrate, protein, fat, vitamins and minerals. However, some nutritional issues deserve particular attention in some categories of disability. In addition, a few practical issues should be considered.

Issues and Solutions

Whilst carbohydrate and protein remain an important part of the athlete's diet, athletes with mobility problems need to take this into account when calculating intakes. Requirements can be reduced to as little as half those required for able bodied athletes, if mobility is severely restricted.

Athletes may need assistance in obtaining food and fluids. Drinks bottles that attach to wheelchairs, camel backs, or similar equipment may help.

Access to toilets may put wheelchair users off drinking enough fluid, but it is vital that all athletes drink enough fluid.

Good hydration will help to prevent urinary tract infections, dehydration will increase them. Whilst those with spinal cord injuries will not sweat below the lesion, the sweat rate above the lesion is increased - possibly as much as six fold. Hydration is therefore very important.

During flights, loosen shoe laces to relieve pressure caused by swelling. Access to toilets can be a problem, so athletes should at least try to minimize dehydration and allow time to recover from dehydration when they arrive abroad, especially before undertaking strenuous training in heat.

Autonomic Dysreflexia is a condition which causes a serious and uncontrolled rise in blood pressure. It usually occurs in individuals with a spinal cord lesion above the T6 level, although it can occur below this level and in individuals with incomplete lesions. It is triggered by stimuli below the lesion such as a full bowel, full bladder, pressure sore, burn, or urinary tract infection. For this reason it is important for susceptible wheelchair athletes to avoid constipation, pressure sores and urinary tract infections. The sudden consumption of large volumes of fluid or drinking excess fluid if it is not being passed away should be avoided. Susceptible individuals should ensure that they work out their fluid strategy carefully with the help of a medic and sports dietitian.

Some athletes will have a reduced ability to detect rises in body temperature. Plans for hydration should be carefully worked out and followed.

Dehydration increases the risk of epilepsy in those who are prone.

Visually impaired athletes may have to adopt different methods of assessing hydration status such as frequency of passing urine, estimating how much urine is being passed (a shorter time than normal being an indicator of dehydration) and the smell of urine, which increases in dehydration as the urine becomes more concentrated.

Key Points

≈ **Carbohydrate is the major fuel for sport in disability sports as well as able bodied sport**

≈ **Quantities eaten may have to be adjusted to take mobility levels into account**

≈ **Protein intakes may also have to be adjusted to take account of mobility**

≈ **Fluid intake and good hydration are, if anything, even more important in disability sport**

≈ **Planning and preparation is vital to ensure accessibility of food, fluids and toilet facilities**

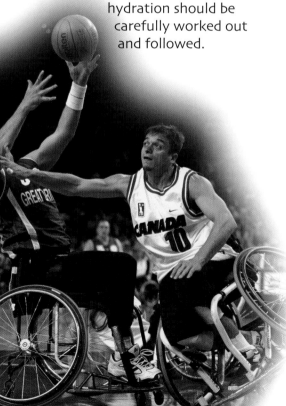

(vii)
Environment Issues
by Jeanette Crosland

Environment affects the nutrition needs of athletes. Competition and training happen in a wide variety of environments including altitude, heat, humidity, cold and pollution. The cold climate is considered in the section on winter sports. Heat and humidity are the environmental factors which can cause the most problems.

Nutrition Issues and Solutions

Fluid loss and the need to replace fluid is the main issue. Fluid requirements can be as high as 10 or more litres a day in hot climates. Whilst not everybody will sweat at this rate, fluid balance is important.

Humidity and heat acclimatization both increase fluid requirements. All athletes should know what their needs are and drink enough to cover them.

Drinks and food must contain enough sodium (salt) to replace that lost through sweat. The addition of salt will help the body to keep more of the fluid inside the body and stimulate thirst - which will increase fluid intake.

Sports drinks containing 4-8% carbohydrate plus sodium are an easy way to provide energy and electrolytes. These provide 160- 320 calories per litre and can increase body weight. Diluted sports drinks plus a pinch of salt, or low calorie squash plus salt might be useful alternatives.

Heat may increase carbohydrate requirements but also reduce appetite. Design and follow a strategy for training and competing in the heat that provides enough carbohydrate as well as fluid.

Competing indoors still involves living in the heat. Drink extra fluid to allow for this.

There is some evidence that altitude and pollution will put the body under extra stress and that antioxidants may be helpful. Eat a varied diet including a wide range of fruit and vegetables plus some sources of vegetable oil to ensure a good intake of antioxidants.

Practical Tips and Ideas

Decide what to drink. This will include different drinks during the day. Work out how much of each is needed

Drinking too much can be as bad as drinking too little

Carry a bottle everywhere and drink regularly

Germs live in dirty drinks bottles so use bottles that can be thrown away after a short time. Alternatively sterilize drinks bottles with sterilizing tablets designed for baby's bottles

Do not share a drinks bottle with anyone

Drink only the drinks you have planned for yourself. Don't take drinks from other people especially in competition and training

Maintain a healthy varied diet including fruit and vegetables - but make sure that fruit is either washed in bottled water or better still peeled

Make sure carbohydrate needs are met

Key Points

≈   Make sure that enough foods containing carbohydrate are eaten

≈   Eat plenty of fruit and vegetables

≈   Drink the amount of fluid that is needed

≈   Consider using a sports drink or adding salt to drinks and food

Know your fluid requirements in different climates. To do this:

≈   Record fluid intake and monitor hydration status. Know the volume of fluid needed to maintain good hydration each day

≈   Use urine testing if scientific support is available

≈   Use the colour of urine to check hydration

≈   Weigh yourself before and after exercise to work out fluid loss. This shows how much fluid is needed for similar sessions

≈   Try not to lose more than about 2% of body weight in a session. Change your drinking strategy to achieve this

≈   Note how often urine is passed in a day - infrequent peeing suggests dehydration

The Diabetic Athlete
by Elaine Hibbert-Jones and Gill Regan

The majority of young people with diabetes will have type 1 diabetes i.e. they require daily insulin injections. Athletes with type 2 diabetes are not discussed here.

Regular physical activity, diet and insulin are the cornerstones of diabetes management. All areas require careful consideration when planning training in order to optimize sporting performance. The young individual in good metabolic control can safely participate in most activities.

Some sports have restrictions and rules concerning athletes with diabetes. National Associations or governing bodies will give advice.

The successful management of blood glucose levels poses a challenge for athletes with diabetes.

It is important to understand how the body regulates its fuels before, during and after exercise in order to successfully manage blood glucose levels. The main areas an athlete needs to consider are:

- *Blood glucose levels*
- *Insulin*
- *Food*

Nutrition Issues and Solutions

Blood glucose control

The body's response to exercise is different in the athlete with diabetes. Balancing blood glucose levels when exercising is a major challenge. Training with either high or low blood glucose levels will make training harder and concentration will be affected. The amount of insulin circulating before, during and after exercise is critical to exercise performance and prevention of fatigue.

- The increased glucose uptake by working muscles may lead to hypoglycaemia (low blood sugar) during exercise

- Too much insulin circulating during exercise also increases blood glucose uptake resulting in hypoglycaemia

- Too little insulin circulating before exercise may cause blood glucose levels to increase and ketones may be present. Exercise can cause the blood glucose levels to go even higher

- Hypoglycaemia can develop some hours after exercise due to the refuelling process where the liver replaces its glycogen stores from circulating glucose in the blood

What should the level of blood glucose be before exercise?

- Avoid exercise if blood glucose level is over 14mmol/l and ketones are present and use caution if over 17mmol/l with no ketones

- Take extra carbohydrate if blood glucose level is under 5.5mmol/l

Diet

- Carbohydrate is the main fuel for working muscles

- A high carbohydrate diet is necessary to ensure good stores of glycogen. Insufficient insulin results in less glycogen being stored. This may affect future training sessions

- The dietary requirements for energy, carbohydrate, protein, fat, vitamins and minerals are no different from a non-diabetic athlete. The skill is to identify when changes in insulin and/or carbohydrate are required to optimize glucose control for training and competition. The athlete should discuss individual insulin and dietary requirements with their diabetes team

Fuelling training and recovery
The amount and type of food needed depends on:

- Pre-exercise blood glucose level

- The frequency, duration and intensity of exercise

- Timing of training sessions

Extra carbohydrate may be needed at four different times:

- 2-3 hours before exercise

- 20-30 mins before exercise

- During exercise

- After exercise

Practical Tips and Ideas

Pre-exercise meal

This should contain a large proportion of starchy carbohydrate e.g. pasta, bread, rice, potatoes, cereals

Pre-exercise/during exercise snack

If needed, choose a carbohydrate snack that suits you e.g. isotonic sports drinks, fruit juice, cereal bar, fresh and dried fruit, confectionery, glucose tablets

Post-exercise snacks

Extra carbohydrate is needed to refuel as well as prevent post-exercise hypos. Suitable snacks include bread, teacakes, cereal bars, muffins, scotch pancakes

Fluid

It is important to drink sufficient fluid before, during and after exercise. Water, low sugar squash, regular squash and isotonic sports drinks can all be useful, depending upon the intensity and duration of the sport and the environment in which it takes place

Key Points

≈ Monitor blood glucose levels before, during and after exercise. Learn your own response to training and competition

≈ Avoid exercise if blood glucose levels are over 14mmol/l with ketones and use caution if over 17mmol/l with no ketones. Take extra carbohydrate if under 5.5mmol/l

≈ Carbohydrate-based foods should be readily available during and after training and competition

≈ Identify when changes in insulin and/or carbohydrate intake are necessary

≈ Keep your hypo remedy available at all times

≈ Discuss your own individual insulin and dietary strategies with your diabetes team

(ix)
The Young and Adolescent Athlete
by Gill Horgan

Like adults, child and adolescent athletes need adequate nutrition to optimize health and performance. Their nutrition must be socially acceptable yet provide for growth and maturation. During periods of growth, active adolescent boys in particular, find it difficult to meet the high energy requirements needed. Puberty in females can lead to a substantial increase in body fat as well as weight and height.

Young athletes are mostly dependent on their parents for their nutrition and mirror the family's eating habits. By the adolescent stage they often develop erratic meal patterns and unbalanced food choices.

Females, in particular, often become preoccupied with restricting energy intake to minimize or reduce changes in body fat levels. Males are more interested in increasing the size and strength of their muscles and often want to try 'body building' type supplements to achieve this. Any dietary advice has to take these concerns into consideration.

Nutrition Issues and Solutions

Energy needs of the growing athlete
During various athletic activities, children use more energy per kg body weight than adolescents and adults.

Protein requirements
Protein needs are greater for children and adolescents than adults. Children aged 7-10 years old need 1.1-1.2g/kg per day and 11-14 year olds need 1g/kg per day. Those who are involved in very intense, regular physical activity may need slightly more than this but in practice most children consume adequate

amounts of protein or even exceed these requirements. However, where there is an element of 'making weight', protein status may not always be optimal, probably due to the restriction of energy intake associated with this practice.

Fluid and electrolyte requirements

Proper hydration is essential for the safety of active children. Children's bodies do not regulate body temperature as efficiently as adults' bodies and are more susceptible to heat injury. Heat injury, usually

Practical Tips and Ideas

Eating foods such as lean meat, poultry, fish, low-fat milk and milk products will provide good sources of protein. If energy intake is adequate to meet the needs for growth and activity, protein requirements will normally be met

Fluid intake should be encouraged before, during and after activity to prevent dehydration. During activity fluids should be encouraged every 15-20 minutes. Drinks containing carbohydrate, sodium and flavour enhance voluntary drinking. The use of dehydration by child athletes to 'make weight' in sports such as wrestling, judo, tae kwon do and boxing should be eliminated

Adolescent athletes who train or compete in the morning, especially those involved in endurance sports, need to eat breakfast. A meal high in carbohydrate could help prevent a premature lowering of blood glucose that occurs if glycogen stores are low after an overnight fast. Those who train or compete during the afternoon or evening should be encouraged to eat and drink 2-3 hours before the exercise session or competition. Foods should be high in carbohydrate; e.g. fruits, juices, breads with jam or honey, breakfast cereals, pasta, or rice

For young athletes who feel nervous before competition, carbohydrate energy bars or fruits are a good alternative. Snacks such as bagels, teacakes, fig rolls, bananas, dried fruit, juice and carbohydrate drinks should also be offered during the day

After exercise, children and adolescents are usually thirsty and hungry and will eat whatever is quickly available. This is a good time to replenish carbohydrate stores

complicated by dehydration, is the second most common sports injury among children, but is the most preventable.

Iron and calcium deficiency
Regular consumption of dairy products is important in ensuring adequate calcium in the diet. Young athletes should aim to eat lean red meat at least three times a week. Alternative food sources of iron include iron-fortified cereals.

A major reason that dietary calcium and iron are low among adolescents is their tendency to shun dairy foods and red meat, either from concern over fat intake or desire for a vegetarian diet.

Key Points

≈ **Take small, frequent meals and snacks which give a balance of nutrients**

≈ **It is beneficial to be well hydrated prior to training and competition. Rule changes may be necessary in some sports to allow for an official 'time out' for players to rehydrate**

≈ **Have a nutritious carbohydrate snack and some fluid after activity to aid refuelling and rehydration**

≈ **If body fat loss is necessary, the first approach should be to adjust food choices so that less fatty foods and snacks are consumed**

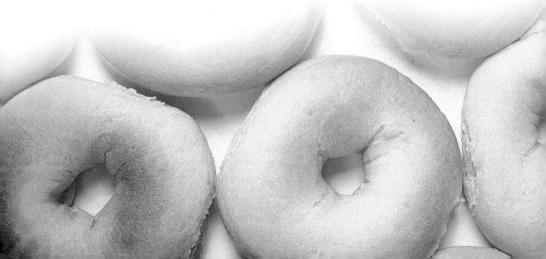

(x)
The Female Athlete
by Jacqueline Boorman

Body composition and weight management are often major dietary concerns in elite athletes. This is particularly true for the female athlete, who despite competing at the highest level may still succumb to the typical pressures placed upon women to achieve a certain body shape. Yet too low a body fat or inadequate energy and carbohydrate intake may result in menstrual irregularities or amenorrhoea (lack of periods), which in-turn may negatively affect bone health e.g. osteopaenia (reduced bone density). However, regular menstruation will result in an increased need for iron in the female athlete - perhaps double or even treble the amount of a non-exercising female.

Nutrition Issues and Solutions

Energy intake

Female athletes should make sure that they eat sufficient energy to meet the demands of their training. Eating a wide variety of foods will help to improve the nutrient density of the diet i.e. ensure iron, calcium and other minerals and vitamins are adequate.

Menstrual irregularities and bone health

An inadequate food intake, perhaps specifically low carbohydrate intake, and not the stress of training may lead to reproductive disorders. It is possible that the hormonal irregularities, which lead to sub-optimal bone health, may be made worse by an inadequate intake of calcium. However, the less severe reproductive disorders may have no menstrual symptoms.

Solutions:

- Medical help should be sought from a sports doctor/gynaecologist with an interest in sport, or a sports dietitian, if periods stop for three months or more

- In cases of pre-occupation with body weight or body fatness seek an assessment by a sports dietitian

- Where there is a cycle of 'binge-guilt-starve-binge', seek the help of a sports dietitian or clinical psychologist

Poor iron status

Whilst true iron-deficiency anaemia is rare in elite athletes, a poor iron store, as reflected in a low ferritin level (below 30µg/l) is common in female athletes. Having a very low iron store will make athletes feel generally fatigued, they may catch frequent infections and fail to recover between training sessions. If an iron supplement is prescribed, ask the doctor or dietitian to suggest an alternative to ferrous sulphate, as this can cause constipation.

Solutions:

- Have an iron-rich diet, and include rich sources of vitamin C to aid iron absorption from plant foods e.g. orange juice, potatoes, kiwi fruit and tomatoes

- Routinely monitor iron stores (serum ferritin) and blood haemoglobin e.g. 2-4 times a year

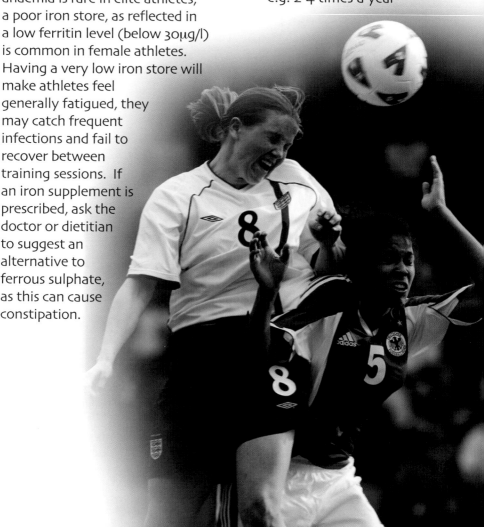

Practical Tips and Ideas

Athletes should ask their coach in advance for training schedules and plan meals and snacks around the training schedule

Keep an honest food and mood diary to develop an understanding of when, what and why food is eaten

Avoid fad diets

Ideally athletes should reflect rationally on their weekly (naked) body-weight alongside food diary records and skinfold measurements if taken

Unless monitoring hydration status, avoid daily weighing

Enjoy iron-rich foods 3-5 times a week such as meat, especially lean red meat e.g. beef, lamb, venison, and oily fish such as salmon, fresh tuna or mackerel

Beans, nuts, eggs and green vegetables are a good source of iron - include these every day, particularly if vegetarian

Drink a glass of orange juice with a meal to enhance iron absorption from plant foods

Eat at least one bowl of iron-fortified breakfast cereal and milk a day - perhaps as a snack?

Try a fruity milkshake, yoghurts or fromage frais as snacks immediately after training as a great source of protein and carbohydrate

Choose low fat dairy products rather than avoiding completely to ensure good calcium nutrition

Key Points

≈ Energy intake must be adequate to meet the demands of training

≈ Extreme weight loss techniques place reproductive and skeletal health as well as performance at risk

≈ Amenorrhoea is not a normal consequence of training, but is a clear sign that health is being compromised

≈ Athletes can prevent reproductive disorders or restore reproductive function through dietary reform without any modification to their training schedule

≈ Ensuring a good intake of iron-rich and calcium-rich foods is particularly important for female athletes

≈ An iron supplement may be prescribed to improve iron stores

≈ Using a food, mood, hunger and exercise diary can help plan meals and snacks

≈ Medical and dietetic opinions should be sought if periods stop or an athlete feels 'out of control' with eating habits and bodyweight

(xi)
The Vegetarian Athlete by Wendy Martinson

A vegetarian diet can be healthy, but athletes following a vegetarian diet need to be aware of the potential nutrient deficiencies that can occur if their diet is not carefully planned.

There are many different variations of the vegetarian diet and most exclude meat products, fish and poultry, but some may include eggs and/or milk and milk products. Vegan diets are very restrictive and exclude all animal foods and products e.g. meat, fish, dairy foods and eggs.

Nutrition Issues and Solutions

Vegetarians
Nutrients that can be lacking from vegetarian diets depend on which foods are excluded. Protein, iron and zinc may be deficient if meat products, poultry, fish and eggs are excluded, plus calcium, riboflavin, vitamin D and vitamin B12 if dairy foods are also excluded. (See section on vitamins and minerals in chapter 6)

Protein
Athletes have a higher requirement for protein and so it is important to ensure that a protein source is included at each meal. Good protein sources are milk, milk products and eggs, pulses (peas e.g. chickpeas and beans e.g. kidney, mung, black eyed, lentils), tofu, textured vegetable/soya protein, Quorn, nuts and nut butters, seeds and seed pastes e.g. tahini. Grains such as rice, bread, pasta, oats and breakfast cereals will also provide protein as well as being a rich source of carbohydrate.

Calcium
Dairy foods are the richest source of calcium, but if these are excluded fortified soya products such as milk, yoghurt, cheese, are an excellent calcium-rich alternative. Other sources of calcium include spinach, broccoli, watercress, spring greens, dried figs, rhubarb, sesame seeds, almonds, brazil nuts and pulses.

Iron

Good sources of iron include pulses, dark green leafy vegetables, seeds, nuts, dried fruits, fortified breakfast cereals, wholemeal bread, whole grains and eggs. To enhance the absorption of iron from plant foods, include a food rich in vitamin C with the meal (e.g. orange juice).

Zinc

Rich sources of zinc are pulses, nuts, seeds, wholegrains, wholemeal bread and eggs.

Vegans

Vegans are also at risk of being deficient in protein, calcium, iron and zinc (see above). In addition, vegans are at risk of deficiencies in vitamins B12, D and riboflavin and rich sources of these should be included in the diet where possible.

Vitamin B12

Vitamin B12 is found in rich supply in animal products, dairy products and eggs. However it can also be found in fortified yeast extract/vegetable stock, fortified soya milk, fortified breakfast cereals and fortified textured vegetable protein.

Riboflavin

Rich sources include yeast extract, wheat germ, fortified breakfast cereals, almonds, soya products, pumpkin, sunflower and sesame seeds.

Vitamin D

Sunlight is the best source! Some foods are fortified with vitamin D such as soya milk, soya cheese and yoghurts, fortified breakfast cereal, vegan margarines e.g. Tomor, Granose.

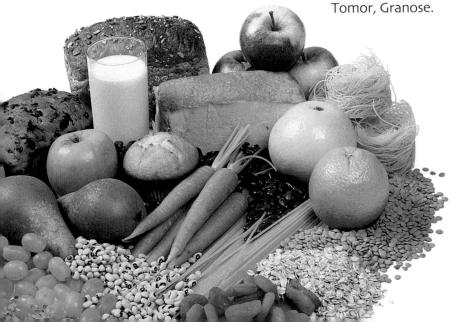

Practical Tips and Ideas

For an excellent recovery drink containing carbohydrate and protein make a smoothie with yoghurt or milk (dairy or fortified soya versions)

Those who do eat dairy foods should choose lower fat varieties to keep fat intake down

Eat large helpings of breakfast cereals in the morning or for snacks to boost iron intake and provide lots of carbohydrate

Increase iron absorption by squeezing vitamin C rich lemon juice on vegetables and pulses or by drinking a glass of fruit juice with the meal

Include nutritious snacks such as dried fruits and nuts, cereal bars, and sandwiches/bagels with hummous, peanut butter or low fat cheese

Key Points

≈ **Plan meals carefully to avoid potential nutrient deficiencies**

≈ **Include plenty of breakfast cereals, bread, rice, pasta and grains to meet carbohydrate needs**

≈ **Include protein-rich foods at each meal e.g. nuts, seeds, pulses, dairy/fortified soya products**

≈ **Include 2-3 servings of fortified soya products every day to provide a calcium-rich alternative to dairy foods**

≈ **Include a vitamin C source with your meal to enhance iron absorption form vegetable foods**

(xii)
The Travelling Athlete
by Penny Hunking

Travelling to competition is part of an athlete's life and it puts weeks and months of hard training to the test. Travelling can involve different forms of transport, delays and even change of time zones, and without intervention, athletes will be limited to the food provided on the way. At the competition venue, the food available will vary. Access to food will change according to the type of accommodation chosen. Some countries have lower standards of food hygiene and athletes must take care with food and drinks to help avoid possible gastrointestinal upsets. With good preparation many of the nutritional challenges posed by travelling can be overcome.

Nutrition Issues and Solutions

Meeting nutritional needs
Getting enough energy, carbohydrate, protein, vitamins and minerals can be difficult, particularly if relying solely on food provided by others.

Meals and snacks may be too high in fat and too low in carbohydrate. Choose wisely in cafes and restaurants.

Always carry snacks and drinks but be careful when travelling to foreign countries as some will not allow travellers to take in certain foods.

Keeping well hydrated
Normal drinking routines can be upset, and air conditioning e.g. on trains and air flights can be dehydrating. Familiar drinks may not be available. Carry appropriate drinks with you at all times.

Getting the quantity right
Travelling can be lengthy, boring and prone to delays so avoid eating for 'something to do'. Plan your eating routines and stick to them.

Food safety
Always choose 'safe' food and drink and never take a chance or you may be put out of competition before you get there! Unpeeled fruit, tap water, ice cubes in drinks, ice cream, sea foods and salads, are the highest risk foods.

Planning and preparation
Find out what food is available at the venue and at your accommodation and plan

strategies to cope. Carry any vital foods with you both for the journey and, if needed, for the duration of your stay.

Find out which foods cannot be taken into the country you are visiting.

Practical Tips and Ideas

To eat: Pack foods that do not require cooking, are sturdy and non-perishable e.g. cereal, muesli and energy bars, powdered milk, breakfast cereals, dried fruit, low fat biscuits, tinned fruit, liquid meal supplements

To drink: Bottled water, sports drinks, long life cartons of milkshake

Accommodation: Book where to stay with meals in mind. Find one that offers suitable meals or book self catering accommodation where you are able to prepare your own meals and snacks

Eating out: Order meals with plenty of potatoes, pasta, rice and cereals and avoid those with added fats especially those that are fried, creamed and sautéed. Ask for extra bread if necessary

Athletes watching body weight: Avoid high fat foods, plan in advance what you will eat and keep to your plan. Don't be influenced by other athletes, boredom or wanting to try new foods

Key Points

≈ **Do your research before you go and find out what food and drink is available whilst travelling and at the venue**

≈ **Try to keep eating and drinking patterns as similar to those practised at home as possible**

≈ **Take familiar food and drink with you if necessary**

≈ **Eat only at reputable cafes and restaurants and drink only bottled water in sealed containers if food safety is questionable**

≈ **Be assertive and ask for something different to eat and drink if necessary. Don't just eat what other athletes are eating, eat to suit you**

≈ **Prepare, plan and pack**

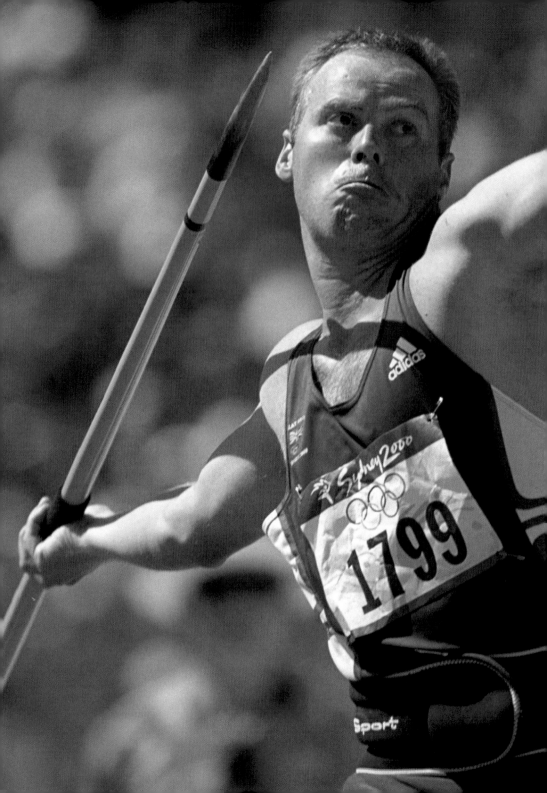

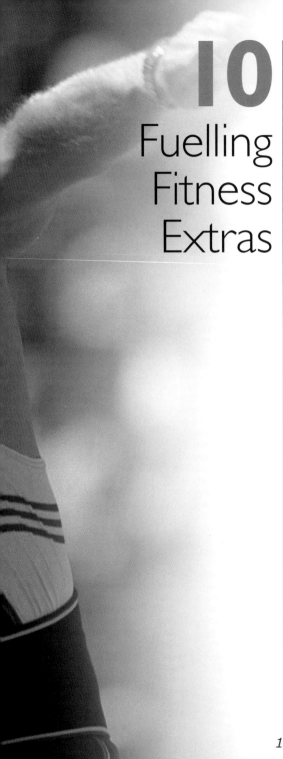

10

Fuelling Fitness Extras

**Jeanette Crosland
and
Penny Hunking**

*Bringing it
All Together ~
Theory into
Practice*

Now you have read the theory it's time to put things into practice! The following section contains lists of foods and their nutrient content and ideas for meals and snacks and what to carry in your kit bag. There's also a log for you to record your own personal food and drink intake to see how well you are fuelling for sports performance.

Meal Ideas

Include plenty of variety in your daily food. Some of the following suggestions might give you some ideas.

Pick and mix the suggestions and choose more or less foods at each meal depending on your appetite and energy requirements.

Breakfast

- Breakfast cereal or porridge and lower fat milk e.g. top with banana, strawberries, cherries, dried apricots or with fresh/dried fruit of your choice

- Cereal such as muesli with low fat yoghurt instead of milk

- Scotch pancakes or crumpets with jam, marmalade or honey

- Scrambled or poached egg or grilled bacon with toast

- Baked beans on toast

- Pancakes cooked in a very hot pan with very little oil topped with syrup and fruit

- Fruit juice

- Bagels or hot cross buns

- Fruit salad with yoghurt

- Fruit smoothie

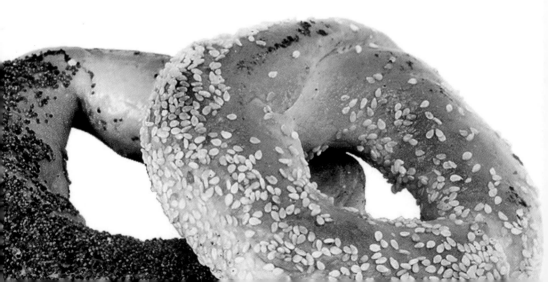

Snack Meals

Sandwiches

- Try different breads e.g. white, brown, granary, high grain, rye
- Include different types of bread e.g. rolls, pitta, soft flour tortillas, French sticks
- Use different fillings e.g. meat, chicken, lower fat cheeses, egg, mashed banana with honey, low fat soft cheese and dates, grilled lean bacon with salad, peanut butter, cottage cheese with fresh or canned fruit added, tuna with low fat mayonnaise and olives
- Serve with a salad

Jacket potatoes

Serve with a variety of fillings such as:

- Cottage cheese with added fresh or canned fruit
- Tuna with sweetcorn and a small amount of low fat mayonnaise or plain yoghurt
- Tinned ratatouille
- Baked beans
- Chilli con carne with meat or a vegetarian version
- Serve with vegetables or salad

Salads

- Prepare with a variety of vegetables including raw mushrooms, mange tout, cauliflower, sweetcorn, peppers, as well as the traditional salad vegetables
- Make salads with cous cous, pasta or rice
- Serve with bread or bread rolls
- Include ready cooked meat, chicken, turkey, tinned fish such as tuna, sardines, salmon, smoked salmon, low fat cheese, cottage cheese, fish fingers, soya or tofu products or boiled egg

Soups

- Ring the changes and choose minestrone, vegetable or meat broth with lentils, beans or barley and serve with extra bread

Hot Meals

TOP TIP: SERVE HOT MEALS WITH PLENTY OF SALAD AND VEGETABLES OF YOUR CHOICE

- Pasta with tomato based sauce and grated cheese
- Jacket potato filled with tuna and sweetcorn or a low fat filling of your choice
- Soup with added pasta, rice or boiled potatoes
- Rice, bean and vegetable stir fry
- Curry e.g. chicken, vegetable, prawn with boiled rice
- Seafood noodles
- Chilli con carne with boiled rice
- Cous cous and roasted Mediterranean vegetables
- Baked beans or sardines on toast
- Mushroom risotto
- Mixed bean pilaf

Desserts

- Apple crumble and low fat ice cream
- Bananas and low fat custard
- Fresh fruit salad
- Bowl of low fat fruit yoghurt
- Low fat rice pudding with jam
- Stuffed baked apples
- Pancakes with lemon juice and sugar
- Summer pudding
- Meringue nest with summer fruits and low fat fromage frais
- Stewed fruit and low fat custard

Kit Bag Snacks

- PUT YOURSELF IN CONTROL OF WHAT YOU EAT AND DRINK
- CARRY SUITABLE SNACKS AND DRINKS IN YOUR KIT BAG

It's vital to have the right food around to eat whenever you need it so don't rely on always being able to buy suitable meals and snacks when you are training or travelling. Put yourself in control and always carry snacks and drinks with you in your kit bag. This needn't be time consuming or complicated, but it does take a little thought. Here are a few ideas of food and drinks that are usually readily available and easily transportable. Of course, if you are travelling around and can't guarantee them being available at your destination, remember to shop for them before you go!

- Bottled water
- Squash
- Isotonic sports drinks
- Cartons of fruit juice

- Low fat yogurt
- Smoothies
- Milkshakes
- Rice pudding
- Pots of custard

- Fresh, dried or tinned fruit
- Bagel
- Muffin
- Scone
- Fruit bread
- Malt loaf
- Scotch pancakes
- Bread sticks
- Cereal bars
- Fruit cake
- Crumpet
- Scone
- Breakfast cereals

- Biscuits e.g. Garibaldi, ginger biscuits, fig roll, digestives, Jaffa cakes
- Rice/pasta, cooked and served cold as a 'salad'

- Jelly beans
- Jelly sweets
- Boiled sweets
- Kendal mint cake

MY PERSONAL FOOD AND DRINK RECORD

To find out how well you are fuelling for sports performance make a chart like this one and complete it as accurately as you can using the tables in this book and the information on food labels to help you calculate your intake.

How to fill in your personal food and drink record:

- Weigh foods if unsure of portion sizes

- Complete this record for as many days as you wish

- Record your food and drink intake on both training days & rest days

- Write down EVERYTHING you eat AND drink

- Keep your record with you and note down what you eat and drink as soon as possible - it is easy to forget!

- Give as much detail as possible e.g. medium slice of white bread, 60g lean ham, 4 dried apricots, 250ml semi-skimmed milk, 1 slice of tomato

Date:					
	Food & drink	How much?	CHO (g)	Protein (g)	Fat (g)
Breakfast					
Snack					
Lunch					
Snack					
Dinner					
Snack					
TOTAL					

Note: CHO stands for carbohydrate

FUELLING FITNESS FOOD CHART

Use these figures, along with those you find on food labels to calculate your daily intake of carbohydrate (CHO), protein and fat.

	Amount g or ml	CHO	Protein	Fat
Fruit				
Apple, eating, average	100	12	0	0
Banana, medium, peeled	100	23	1	0
Dried apricots	100	36	4	1
Grapes	100	15	0	0
Orange, medium	160	14	2	0
Pear, medium	150	16	0	0
Pineapple, thick slice	80	8	0	0
Raisins	100	70	3	1
Tin of fruit salad in juice	410	50	1	0
Tomato, raw, medium	85	3	1	0
Vegetables				
Broccoli, boiled	85	1	3	1
Carrots, young, boiled	60	3	0	0
Green/French beans, boiled	90	3	2	1
Peas, boiled	70	7	5	1
Potato, baked, old, flesh & skin, medium	180	57	7	0
Potato, boiled	175	30	3	0
Sweetcorn, canned, reheated, drained	850	23	2	1

Note: All figures are rounded to the nearest whole number.

	Amount g or ml	CHO	Protein	Fat
Rice & Pasta				
Cous Cous	140	77	9	2
Egg noodles, boiled	230	30	5	1
Pasta, various, boiled	200	64	13	3
Rice, brown, boiled	180	58	5	2
Rice, white, boiled	180	53	4	1
Spaghetti, white, boiled	220	49	8	2
Dairy Foods				
Cheddar cheese, average	40	0	10	14
Cottage cheese, plain, reduced fat	112	4	15	2
Ice cream, dairy, vanilla	75	19	3	7
Milk, skimmed	200	10	6	0
Milk, semi-skimmed	200	10	6	2
Milk, whole	200	10	6	8
Yoghurt, drinking	200	26	6	0
Yoghurt, low fat, plain	150	11	8	1
Yoghurt, whole milk, plain	150	12	9	5
Breakfast Cereals				
Branflakes	30	21	3	1
Cornflakes	30	26	2	0
Muesli	50	33	6	4
Porridge, milk & water	160	18	5	5
Weetabix	20	15	2	1

Note: All figures are rounded to the nearest whole number.

	Amount g or ml	CHO	Protein	Fat
Beans & Pulses				
Baked beans, canned in tomato sauce	135	20	6	0
Butterbeans, canned, reheated	120	16	7	1
Chickpeas, canned, reheated, drained	35	6	3	1
Lentils, boiled	40	7	3	0
Breads, Biscuits & Cakes				
Bagel	70	39	1	7
Brown, average, medium slice	36	16	3	1
Currant bread, slice	35	18	3	3
Crumpet, fresh	40	15	2	0
Muffin	68	34	7	4
Scone, fruit	48	25	4	5
White, average, medium slice	30	15	3	1
Croissant	60	23	5	12
Danish pastry	110	56	6	19
Doughnut, ring	30	28	4	13
Flapjack	70	42	3	19
Jaffa cake, 1 cake	13	9	0	1
Oat cake biscuit	13	8	1	2
Rye crispbread	10	7	1	0

Note: All figures are rounded to the nearest whole number.

	Amount g or ml	CHO	Protein	Fat
Breads, Biscuits & Cakes				
Battenberg, slice	32	16	2	6
Cheese cake, slice	120	30	4	43
Chocolate cake, slice	40	20	3	11
Madeira cake, slice	40	24	2	7
Egg, Chicken, Meat & Seafood				
Egg, whole, raw	61	0	8	7
Chicken breast, grilled, meat only	130	0	42	3
Beef, fillet steak, raw, lean	142	0	30	9
Ham, slice	23	0	4	1
Pork, steak, raw, lean	100	0	22	3
Sausage, pork, grilled, medium	20	2	3	4
Salmon, grilled	82	0	20	11
Tuna, canned in brine	100	0	24	1
Nuts & Seeds				
Cashews, plain	10	2	2	5
Peanuts, plain	13	2	3	6
Sunflower seeds	16	3	3	8

Note: All figures are rounded to the nearest whole number.

	Amount g or ml	CHO	Protein	Fat
Spreads				
Honey	17	13	0	0
Marmalade	15	10	0	0
Stonefruit jam	15	10	0	0
Peanut butter, wholegrain	20	2	5	11
Mayonnaise	30	1	0	23
Fats & Oils				
Butter	10	0	1	8
Margarine	10	0	0	8
Olive oil	11	0	0	11
Confectionery				
Boiled sweets (each)	7	6	0	0
Fruit gums/jelly (tube)	40	32	3	0
Fruit pastilles (tube)	40	25	2	0
Turkish delight (one piece)	15	12	0	0
Fudge (one piece)	11	9	0	2
Milk chocolate standard bar	50	28	4	15
Plain chocolate standard bar	50	32	3	14
Chocolate covered wafer fingers (4 fingers)	50	32	4	13

Note: All figures are rounded to the nearest whole number.

	Amount g or ml	CHO	Protein	Alcohol
Drinks				
Isotonic sports drink	500	30	0	0
Orange juice	200	18	1	0
Carrot juice	50	3	0	0
Grape juice	160	19	0	0
Mango juice (canned)	160	23	0	0
Blackcurrant juice drink (diluted)	288	23	0	0
Lime juice cordial (undiluted)	45	13	0	0
Orange drink (undiluted)	50	14	0	0

Note: All figures are rounded to the nearest whole number. The drink examples do not contain fat so calorie content from alcohol is shown instead

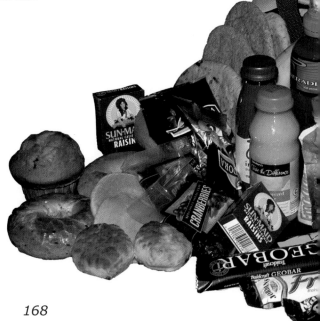

	Amount g or ml	CHO	Protein	Alcohol
Drinks				
Lemonade (can)	343	20	0	0
Cola (can)	343	37	0	0
Beer bitter (1 pint)	568	13	2	16
Lager (1 pint)	568	14	2	23
Red wine (small glass)	125	0	0	12
White wine (small glass)	125	4	0	11
Spirits 40% alcohol (pub measure)	35	0	0	11

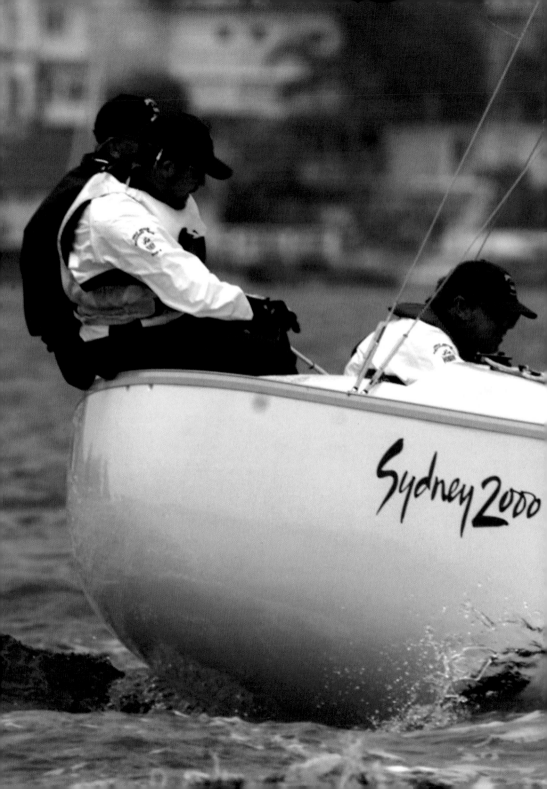

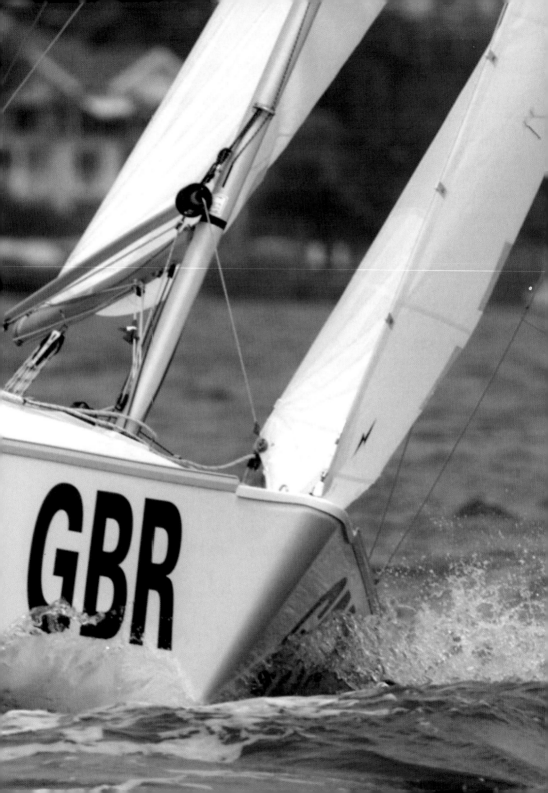

References

Fuelling Fitness for Sports Performance is based on the conclusions of the International Olympic Committee (IOC) Consensus Conference on Sports Nutrition, Lausanne, June 2003.

The full manuscripts from the Consensus Conference have been published as a Special Issue of the Journal of Sports Sciences, January 2004 (ISSN: 2064-0414):

Loucks A.B. (2004). Energy balance and body composition in sports and exercise. *Journal of Sports Sciences* **22**: 1-14.

Burke L.M., Kiens B. and Ivy J.L. (2004). Carbohydrates and fat for training and recovery. *Journal of Sports Sciences* **22**: 15-30.

Hargreaves M., Hawley J.A. and Jeukendrup A. (2004). Pre-exercise carbohydrate and fat ingestion: effects on metabolism and performance. *Journal of Sports Sciences* **22**: 31-38.

Coyle E.F. (2004). Fluid and fuel intake during exercise. *Journal of Sports Sciences* **22**: 39-55.

Shirreffs S.M., Armstrong L.E. and Cheuvront S.N. (2004). Fluid and electrolyte needs for preparation and recovery from training and competition. *Journal of Sports Sciences* **22**: 57-63.

Tipton K.D. and Wolfe R.R. (2004). Protein and amino acids for athletes. *Journal of Sports Sciences* **22**: 65-79.

Powers S.K., DeRuisseau K.C., Quindry J. and Hamilton K.L. (2004). Dietary antioxidants and exercise. *Journal of Sports Sciences* **22**: 81-94.

Maughan R.J., King D.S. and Lea T. (2004). Dietary supplements. *Journal of Sports Sciences* **22**: 95-113.

Gleeson M., Nieman D.C. and Pedersen B.K. (2004). Exercise, nutrition and immune function. *Journal of Sports Sciences* **22**: 115-125.

Spriet L.L. and Gibala M.J. (2004). Nutritional strategies to influence adaptations to training. *Journal of Sports Sciences* **22**: 127-141.

The IOC Consensus papers are also available as a book:

**Nutrition for Athletes. Edited by R.J. Maughan, L.M. Burke
and E.F. Coyle (2004).** ISBN 0-415-33906-5 Routledge.

Suggested Further Reading:

**Handbook of Sports Medicine and Science: Sports Nutrition.
Edited by R.J. Maughan and L.M. Burke (2002).** An IOC Medical
Commission Publication.
ISBN 0-632-05814-5 Blackwell Publishing.

**Manual of Dietetic Practice (Third edition).
Edited by B. Thomas (2001).**
ISBN 0-632-05524-3 Blackwell Publishing.

**McCance and Widdowson's the Composition of Foods: Summary
Edition (2002).**
ISBN 0-854-04428-0 Royal Society of Chemistry.

The Diabetic Athlete. S. Colberg (2001).
ISBN 0-7360-3271-1 Human Kinetics.

**The Encyclopedia of Sports Medicine. Volume VII: Nutrition in
Sport. Edited by R.J. Maughan (2000).**
An IOC Medical Commission Publication in collaboration with the
International Federation of Sports Medicine.
ISBN 0-632-05094-2 Blackwell Publishing.

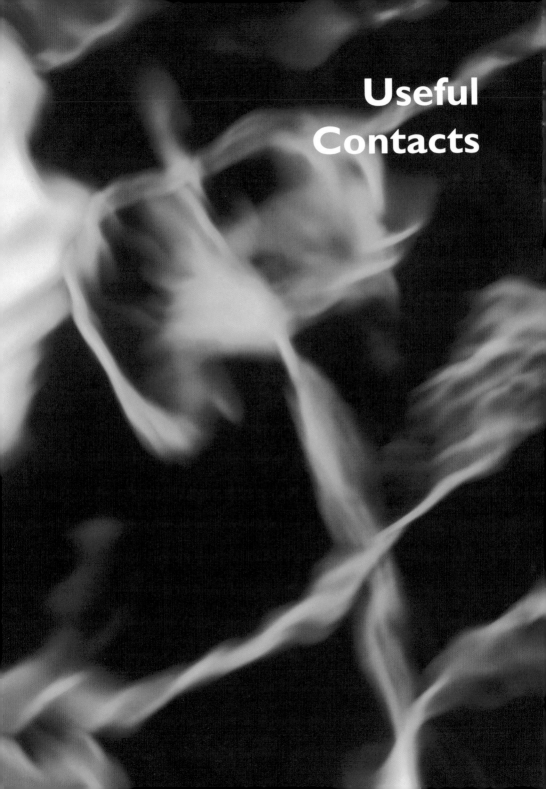

Useful
Contacts

British Dietetic Association
5th Floor
Charles House
148/9 Great Charles Street
Queensway
Birmingham B3 3HT
www.bda.uk.com

British Olympic Association
1 Wandsworth Plain
London SW18 1ET
www.olympics.org.uk

British Paralympic Association
9th Floor Norwich Union Building
69 Park Lane
Croydon
Surrey CR9 1BG
www.paralympics.org.uk

Dietitians in Sport and Exercise
Nutrition (DISEN)
PO Box 22360
London W13 9FL
www.disen.org

Diabetes UK
10 Parkway
London NW1 7AA
www.diabetesuk.co.uk

Eating Disorders Association
103 Prince of Wales Road
Norwich NR1 1DW
www.edauk.com

National Osteoporosis Society
Camerton
Bath BA2 0PJ
www.nos.org.uk

Nutrition Society
10 Cambridge Court
210 Shepherds Bush Road
London W6 7NJ
www.nutritionsociety.org

Olympic Medical Institute
Northwick Park Hospital
Watford Road
Harrow
Middlesex HA1 3UJ
www.olympics.org.uk/omi

Sports Coach UK
114 Cardigan Road
Headingley
Leeds LS6 3BJ
www.sportscoachuk.org

The Sugar Bureau
Duncan House
Dolphin Square
London SW1V 3PW
www.sugar-bureau.co.uk

UK Sport
40 Bernard Street
London WC1N 1ST
www.uksport.gov.uk

World Anti-Doping Agency
(WADA)
European Office
Avenue du Tribunal-Fédéral 34
1005 Lausanne
Switzerland
www.wada-ama.org